W9-ABM-535

Springer Series on _____
ADULTHOOD and AGING

Series Editor: Bernard D. Starr, Ph. D.

Advisory Board: Paul D. Baltes, Ph. D. Jack Botwinick, Ph. D., Carl Eisdorfer, M.D., Ph.D.,Robert Kastenbaum, Ph. D., Neil G. McCluskey, Ph. D., K. Warner Schaie, Ph. D., and Nathan W. Shock, Ph. D.

Harold J. Wershow, D.S.W., is Professor of Sociology in
the Department of Sociology, University College, The
University of Alabama in Birmingham. He taught there
for nineteen years after fifteen years as a social worker
with foster children, families, and the chronically ill and
aged. He received his B.S. degree from City College of
New York with honors in social science, and his masters
and doctoral degrees from the School of Social Work,
University of Pennsylvania. He is a fellow of the Gerontological Society and a member of the American Sociological Association, Sigma Xi Honorary Scientific Society,
and the National Association of Social Workers. He was
Fulbright–Hayes Lecturer to the School of Social Work,
Haifa University, Israel in 1977–78, and visiting scholar
in the Agricultural University of The Netherlands at
Wageningen in 1974–75. His publications include papers
on aging in the kibbutz, priority-setting in health and
welfare services, and problems of statistical data on aging.

CONTROVERSIAL ISSUES IN GERONTOLOGY

Harold J. Wershow, Editor
with Contributors

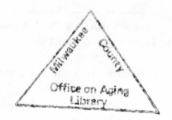

SPRINGER PUBLISHING COMPANY
New York

86- 911

Springer Publishing Company, Inc.
200 Park Avenue South
New York, New York   10003

81 82 83 84 85 / 10 9 8 7 6 5 4 3 2 1

Library of Congress Cataloging in Publication Data
Main entry under title:

Controversial issues in gerontology.

    (Springer series on adulthood and aging; 10)
    Bibliography: p.
    Includes index.
    1. Gerontology—United States—Addresses, essays,
lectures.   I. Wershow, Harold J.   II. Series.
[DNLM: 1. Aging.   2. Geriatrics.   W1 SP685N v.   10 / WT
104 C764]
HQ1064.U5C612   305.2'6   81-1988
ISBN 0-8261-3100-X   AACR2
ISBN 0-8261-3101-8 (pbk.)

Printed in the United States of America

To

Al Goldfarb

and

Art Waldman

pioneers in realistic research and service to the aged

May their memories

be for us a blessing

Contents

PART FOUR   CULTURAL AND SOCIAL DIMENSIONS

PART FIVE   POLICY AND SERVICE ISSUES

PART SIX   A POTPOURRI OF ISSUES

PART SEVEN   EPILOGUE

Foreword

It is a pleasure to write a foreword for a book that, had I thought of it in time, I might have tried to develop myself. My early enthusiasm for Harold Wershow's idea of explicating controversy within gerontology became even greater when I was able to peruse the final version. Controversy and conflict are required for growth in any field.

For many years gerontologists have had to defend the significance of their work and the importance of their community of interests. They were accused of displaying morbid interests, of serving as advocates for persons whose futurity was limited and thus of limited value, of caring for people who didn't matter. Gerontologists are familiar with these controversies: controversies about the meaningfulness of their endeavors, about the pertinence of their research and service efforts.

Now the wheel of fortune has turned. It is the advocates of the young, of children and public schools and child care centers, who are complaining that their pleas are going unheard. I'm not arguing that the elderly are uniformly well-off, but that in recent turns of the wheel, they have fared better on the whole than other age groups and population groups. Certainly, to the extent that support can be measured by media portrayal, the elderly are well-supported. The books, articles, educational films, academic journals, and general media mentions of aging and the elderly have grown, first to a stream and, now, to a river torrent. There is no doubt: "Aging" is in. That doesn't equate to "old people got it good," but it does mean that they have lots of attention and verbalized support.

In spite of gerontology's recent acceptance, controversy within the field has not been especially important, except for the chronic, often boring and irrelevant debate over disengagement theory. And this has become less a fruitful debate than an attempt to bury a mutilated body before it had been fully tested for signs of life. In bringing into focus the more significant controversies within the field, Wershow is providing further evidence that gerontology, which I view as a series of subspecialities linked together by concern for the later years of life, is now coming of age.

As gerontologists, we have now been admitted to the sanctuary of the acceptables. We can stop defending ourselves and attend to the controversies and untested assumptions that exist within our own fields. We can look to our heresies and see what we can learn from them, always remaining vigilant that yesterday's heresies not become tomorrow's platitudinous truisms.

It is difficult for advocates, whether their advocacy is expressed through service or through research, to be impartial about the general worthiness of those for whom they stand advocate. Nor is there any need that they should. I would personally wonder about a gerontologist who found it troublesome to be with older people or who took a stance of total objectivity about their concerns. Nonetheless, there is a strong tendency to view those for whom we advocate as the repository of many more virtues than actually adhere. We attempt to retain perspective by claiming that "of course, some older people aren't like that," but our tone implies that the only older people who are not virtuous, wise, and wonderful are those who have been so distorted by society that their imperfections are hardly their own doing, although their perfections are completely so.

Older people are, first and foremost, people. They have all the wonderful, terrible, beautiful, ugly, sexual, nonsexual, creative, stultifying, growing, limiting, abandoned, constricted qualities that appear among all age groups. Wisdom does not automatically accrue with age; wisdom accrues with a person's experiences and how that person integrates and acts upon the experiences. It may be extremely difficult to be wise without being experienced, and it may be extremely difficult to be experienced without having lived long enough to have experiences, and it may therefore be true that older persons have more than their share of wisdom, but it isn't automatically conferred.

In pursuing the idea that older people are people, it follows for me that they are neither reprehensible nor cute when they express their sexual desires, their artistic competence, or their needs for personal intimacy. We—and gerontologists are as guilty as others—smile benignly at an elderly couple holding hands, much as we do when 10-year-olds hold hands; we wink knowingly, confirming our permission to go ahead, when we hear of sexually active older persons. Older people may need to be recognized as human beings with rights and responsibilities equal to all other adult human beings, but they don't need our permission to be who they are. It's equally all right for any older person to avoid sex altogether, if that individual so prefers.

So older people have more of this and less of that, and what they have more of may be less valued by society and what they have less of may be more valued by society, but these values did not develop in order to punish older people. And, in fact, today's older people were perpetrators of these values long before they were victims. But the elderly are not qualitatively different than the nonelderly. They are merely quantitatively different with regard to certain characteristics, and even that may be limited to this period of history.

However, being quantitatively different is not without meaning. While we must attend to immense individual differences among older persons, we cannot ignore some of the conspicuous trends. Thus, many more older people have lost a spouse through death, have suffered hearing or visual losses, have diminished income, and anticipate relatively brief futurity. When we plan for large groups of older persons, these characteristics must be taken into account; when we view an individual older person, we must avoid assuming too much too soon. Unfortunately, we are caught in a classical bind: as we are evaluating our assumptions, we must also act, and sometimes our assumptions are all that we have on which to base decisions.

I believe that I share many of Wershow's personal biases. We both appear to believe that too many assumptions about older persons are screened through the biased lenses of middle-class, middle-aged viewers, supported by a small cadre of older persons who aggressively share their views and visions. For example, I personally believe that tomorrow's elderly will rue the changes in mandatory retirement regulations, not because the changes were inappropriate, but because I anticipate changes in social security and retirement benefits to be tied to the new retirement age. I also recall the pride with which one outreach worker described her successful efforts in pressuring some very old men to apply for benefits to which they were entitled, ignoring their initial claims that their sense of well-being rested partly on their ability to live without welfare, especially since their ethnic community deprecated welfare recipients. They had not sought her counsel, nor did they ever thank her, and I believe their loss of pride was too great a price for their food stamps and welfare checks. But these last two descriptions represent assumptions of mine, untested and requiring the same rigorous examination as the assumptions that they attack.

One last point. Both research investigators and service-providers need to develop awareness of and respect for each other's sources of knowledge, while retaining a healthy skepticism for their own sources of knowledge. Rigorous, critical thinking is not the province only of the researcher; sensitive, understanding feeling is not the province only of the service-provider. Stereotypes need ferreting out in these regards also.

Both rigor and sensitivity, both thinking and feeling, are required to move past platitudes and to gain knowledge and understanding of what is happening and of what is changing.

So many thanks to Harold Wershow for providing these views of controversy and heresy. This book is a harbinger of exciting days ahead in gerontology.

Richard A. Kalish, Ph.D.

Acknowledgments

Anonymous. "Case Conference: . . . Strive Officiously to Keep Alive?" Reprinted
from *Journal of Medical Ethics* 3 (1977) by permission.
Arie, T. "Brain Failure in Old Age: Thoughts on Rationing and Responsibility." In
W. F. Anderson and J. R. Carlton-Ashton (Eds.), *Brain Failure in Old Age*.
(*Age and Ageing* Supplementary Issue) 6 (1977):104–107. Copyright 1977 by
Baillière Tindall. Reprinted by permission.
Baltes, Paul B. and Schaie, K. Warner. "Aging and IQ: The Myth of the Twilight
Years." Reprinted from *Psychology Today Magazine*, March 1974, pp. 35–
40. Copyright © 1974 Ziff-Davis Publishing Company.
Beeson, Diane. "Women in Studies of Aging: A Critique and Suggestions." *Social
Problems* 23 (October 1975):52–59. Copyright 1975 by the Society for the
Study of Social Problems. Reprinted with permission.
Binstock, Robert. "Federal Policy toward the Aged: Its Inadequacies and its
Politics." *National Journal*, 11 November 1978, pp. 1837–45. Copyright
1978 by Government Research Corporation. Reprinted by permission.
Brocklehurst, J. "Brain Failure in Old Age: Social Implications." In W. F. Anderson
and J. R. Carlton-Ashton (Eds.), *Brain Failure in Old Age*. (*Age and Ageing*
Supplementary Issue) 6 (1977):30–34, 36–40. Copyright 1977 by Baillière
Tindall. Reprinted by permission.
Chadwick, T. "Review of *The Honorable Elders*." *The Gerontologist* 16 (1976):560–
61. Copyright 1976 by the Gerontological Society. Reprinted by permission.
Chaiffetz, Mamie. Anecdote. *The Gerontologist* 8 (1968), 244. Reprinted by per-
mission.
Cook, Fay and Cook, Thomas D. "Evaluating the Rhetoric of Crisis: A Case Study of
Criminal Victimization of the Elderly." *Social Service Review* 50 (December
1976):632–46. Copyright 1976 by the University of Chicago Press. Reprinted
by permission.
———. "Criminal Victimization of the Elderly: Is the Crisis Rhetoric Warranted
Yet?" Original contribution, 1979.
Denes, Magda. *In Necessity and Sorrow: Life and Death in an Abortion Hospital*.
New York: Penguin Books, 1976.

Friday, Paul C. "Sanctioning in Sweden: An Overview." *Federal Probation* 40 (September 1976) 48–55. Administrative Office of United States Courts, in cooperation with Bureau of Prisons, United States Department of Justice. Reprinted by permission.

Goddard, J. "Extension of the Lifespan: A National Goal?" In B. Neugarten and R. Havighurst (Eds.), *Extending the Human Life Span: Social Policy and Social Ethics*. Washington, D.C.: National Science Foundation, 1977.

Havighurst, R. and Sacher, G. "Prospects of Lengthening Life and Vigor." In B. Neugarten and R. Havighurst (Eds.), *Extending the Human Life Span: Social Policy and Social Ethics*. Washington, D.C.: National Science Foundation, 1977. Reprinted by permission.

Hayflick, L. "Perspectives on Human Longevity." In B. Neugarten and R. Havighurst (Eds.), *Extending the Human Life Span: Social Policy and Social Ethics*. Washington, D.C.: National Science Foundation, 1977.

Hochschild, Arlie R. "Disengagement Theory: A Critique and Proposal." *American Sociological Review* 40 (1975):553–59. Copyright 1975 by the American Sociological Association. Reprinted by permission.

Horn, John L. and Donaldson, G. "On the Myth of Intellectual Decline in Aging." *American Psychologist* 31 (1976):701–9. Copyright 1976 by the American Psychological Association. Reprinted by permission.

Hudson, R. "Death, Dying and the Zealous Phase." *Annals of Internal Medicine* 88 (1978):696–702. Copyright 1978 by *Annals of Internal Medicine*. Reprinted by permission.

Kalish, Richard A. "Of Social Values and the Dying: A Defense of Disengagement." *Family Coordinator* (January 1972) pp. 81–94. Copyright 1972 by the National Council on Family Relations. Reprinted by permission.

———. "The New Ageism and the Failure Models: A Polemic." *The Gerontologist* 19 (1979):398–407. Reprinted by permission.

Kline, Chrysee. "The Socialization Process of Women: Implications for a Theory of Successful Aging." *The Gerontologist* 15 (1975):486–92. Copyright 1975 by the Gerontological Society. Reprinted by permission.

Leaf, Alexander. "Every Day Is a Gift When You Are over 100." *National Geographic* (January 1973) pp. 93–117. Copyright 1973 by the National Geographic Society. Reprinted by permission.

———. "Statement Regarding the Purportedly Longevous Peoples of Vilcabamba." Privately reproduced, n.d. Reprinted with permission.

Malinchak, Alan A. and Wright, Douglas. "The Scope of Victimization of the Elderly." *Aging* 281–282 (March-April 1978):12–16. Reprinted by permission.

Martin, Cora A. "Lavender Rose or Gray Panther?" *Aging* 285–286 (July-August 1978):28–30. Reprinted by permission.

McCord, A. "Review of *The Honorable Elders*." *Sociology* 3 (February 1976):69. Reprinted by permission.

Medvedev, Zhores. "Caucasus and Altay Longevity: A Biological or Social Problem?" *Gerontologist* 14 (1974):381–87. Copyright 1974 by the Gerontological Society. Reprinted by permission.

Osmond, Humphrey and Siegler, Miriam. "The Dying Role—Its Clinical Importance." *Alabama Journal of Medical Sciences* 13 (1976):313–17. Reprinted by permission.

Palmore, Erdman. "Facts on Aging: A Short Quiz." *Gerontologist* 17 (1977):315–20. Copyright 1978 by the Gerontological Society. Reprinted by permission.

———. "What Can the USA Learn from Japan about Aging?" *Gerontologist* 15 (1975):64–7. Copyright 1975 by the Gerontological Society. Reprinted by permission.

Riley, M. "Review of *The Honorable Elders*" *Social Forces* 55 (1976):564–65. Reprinted by permission.

Rosow, I. "The Aged in Post-Affluent Society." *Gerontology* (Israel) 1 (1975):9–22. Reprinted by permission.

———. "Retirement Leisure and Social Status," In *Proceedings*. Duke University Council on Aging and Human Development, 1969, 249–257. Reprinted by permission.

Strehler, Bernard L. "A New Age for Aging." *Natural History Magazine* (February 1973) pp. 9–18, 82–5. Copyright © the American Museum of Natural History, 1973. Reprinted with permission.

Tobin, Sheldon S. and Thompson, Dan. "The 'Countability' Paradox of Social Programs." Paper presented at the Xth International Congress of Gerontology, Jerusalem, Israel, June 22–27, 1975. Reprinted by permission.

Wershow, Harold J. "Comment: Reality Orientation for Gerontologists—Some Thoughts about Senility." *Gerontologist* 17 (1977):297–302. Copyright 1977 by the Gerontological Society. Reprinted by permission.

Wilensky, Harold L. "The Politics of Taxation: America in World Perspective." In C. Break and B. Wallin (Eds.), *Taxation: Myth and Realities*. Menlo Park, Calif. and Reading, Mass.: Addison-Wesley, 1978. Copyright © 1978 by the Regents of the University of California. This article was originally written for the Ninth Course by Newspaper, "Taxation: Myths and Realities." Courses by Newspaper is a project of University Extension, University of California, San Diego, and is funded by the National Endowment for the Humanities. Reprinted by permission.

Personal Acknowledgments

Sincerely acknowledged is the assistance of many colleagues, too many to name, who generously aided in the development of this volume by suggesting papers for inclusion. For some, the aid was not in their personal self-interest, as they themselves had either completed or were working on their own anthologies and readers. Also acknowledged here is the aid of Dr. Shlomo Sharlin, Dean of the School of Social Work at Haifa University, who gave me the opportunity to use a portion of my Fulbright year with Haifa University to develop the basic ideas used herein. I am also grateful to Dr. Harold W. Schnaper, Director of the Center on Aging of the University of Alabama in Birmingham, who not only made funds available to have the manuscript prepared, but who gave his warm assent to this effort, and to the successive generations of secretaries, typists, CETA workers, and work-study students who labored faithfully on successive drafts of the manuscript, Ms. Stephanie Small, Ms. Shirley Cotman, Ms. Jane Jacobs, Ms. Christy Kinnaird, and especially to Ms. Dana King. I am also deeply indebted to the authors and publishers who permitted the use of their works, and to Dr. Ursula Springer, Publisher, Dr. Bernard Starr, Editor of the Adulthood and Aging Series, and to the Springer staff, who labored most professionally to produce this book. Last but most of all, I am grateful to my wife, Jean, who uncomplainingly shared our life with my taskmaster, this volume.

Contributors

THOMAS H. ARIE, B.M., B.Che. (Oxford 1950), is Professor of Health Care of the Elderly and Consultant Psychiatrist to Nottingham Hospitals and University of Nottingham. He is a member of the Royal College of Physicians and Central Council of Education of Social Workers, among many other consultancies and boards, and author of many papers in geriatric psychiatry.

PAUL B. BALTES, Ph.D. (University of the Saarland, West Germany 1967), is Professor of Human Development and Director of Individual and Family Studies, Pennsylvania State University. He is author of *Longitudinal and Cross Sectional Sequences in the Study of Age* and numerous papers in the area of intellectual functioning of the aged.

DIANE BEESON, Ph.D. candidate, is Assistant Professor, Graduate Program in Sociology, University of California, San Francisco, and author of papers relating largely to the role of women and prenatal diagnosis.

ROBERT BINSTOCK, Ph.D. (Harvard, 1965), is Stulberg Professor of Law and Politics and Director of the Program in the Politics and Economics of Aging at Brandeis University. He was Executive Director of the White House Task Force on Older Americans under President Johnson, a past president of the Gerontological Society and co-author of the *Handbook of Aging and the Social Sciences*.

JOHN BROCKLEHURST, M.D. (University Hospital of South Manchester, Glasgow, 1950), is Professor of Geriatric Medicine, University of Manchester. Author of *Incontinence in Old People* and *The Geriatric Day Hospital,* among other works.

TERRY B. CHADWICK, M.A. (Portland State University, 1977), is a Ph.D. candidate at Oregon State University. She has had extensive experiences in various projects in aging in Community Action Agency, Gray Panthers, housing for the elderly and community planning, plus study in Egypt and Tunisia.

FAY COOK, Ph.D. (University of Chicago, 1977) is Assistant Professor of Education and Urban Affairs, Northwestern University. Formerly a social worker and teacher of English and social work and author of *Who Should be Helped? Public Support for Social Services,* Dr. Cook is co-author with Thomas Cook and others of *Criminal Victimization of the Elderly.*

THOMAS COOK, Ph.D. (Stanford, 1967) is Professor of Psychology, Northwestern University. Dr. Cook's research interest is in the persistence of induced attitude change and in evaluation research and he is co-author of *Sesame Street Revisited, Criminal Victimization of the Elderly,* and *Qualitative and Quantitative Methods in Evaluation.*

ELAINE CUMMING, Ph.D. (Harvard, 1954), is Professor and Chair, Department of Sociology and Anthropology, University of British Columbia. After beginning her career as a geneticist and cytologist, she became an epidemiologist with the New York State Department of Mental Health. She served on the Provincial (British Columbia) Royal Commission on Aging and Family Life and the National Opinion Research Center and has co-authored *Closed Ranks, Growing Old,* and *Ego and Milieu.*

PAUL C. FRIDAY, Ph.D. (University of Wisconsin, 1970), is Professor of Sociology in Western Michigan University. He has conducted extensive research in criminology in several European countries, as well as the U.S., and has published papers in journals in Sweden, Germany, Italy, and the U.S. He is president of the International Sociological Association's Section on Deviance and Control and a member of the Research Council. He was a Fulbright-Hayes lecturer in Sweden in 1975 and the author of many papers and chapters, including co-editor (with Lorne Stewart) of *Youth Crime and Juvenile Justice.*

JAMES GODDARD, M.D. (George Washington University, 1944), MPH (Harvard, 1955), is a consultant to various food and drug concerns with Alega Associates. His long and distinguished career in public health includes a stint as commissioner of the (Federal) Food and Drug Administration (1966–68).

ROBERT HAVIGHURST, Ph.D. (Ohio State University, 1924), is Professor Emeritus of Human Development, Psychology and Education, University of Chicago, and is a past president of the Gerontological Society, of which he is a founding father. His publications include *Growing Up in River City* and *Adjustment to Retirement.*

LEONARD HAYFLICK, Ph.D. (University of Pennsylvania, 1956), is an associate member of the Western Institute of Philadelphia, Pennsylvania and a consultant to the World Health Organization. Dr. Hayflick is a past president of the Gerontological Society and is discoverer of the agent causing a primary form of atypical pneumonia and the finiteness of life at the cellular level.

ARLIE HOCHSCHILD, Ph.D. (University of California, Berkeley, 1969), is Associate Professor of Sociology, University of California at Berkeley. She is editor of a special issue on women for *Transactions* and of *The Unexpected Community.*

JOHN HORN, Ph.D. (University of Illinois, 1968), is Professor of Psychology, University of Denver and Co-director, Institute of Personality and Ability Testing, Western Branch, Boulder, Colorado. He is author of *Life Span Developmental Psychology.*

ROBERT HUDSON, M.D. (University of Kansas, 1952), is Associate Professor of Medicine and of The History of Medicine at the University of Kansas and an extensive author in the areas of medical history and medical ethics.

RICHARD A. KALISH, Ph.D. (Case-Western Reserve University, 1957), is Professor, California School of Professional Psychology in Berkeley. His major research areas are gerontology and thanatology and he is author of *Death and Ethnicity* and *Death, the Process of Dying and Grief.*

CHRYSEE KLINE was an exceptionally promising graduate student at the School of Social Work, University of Pennsylvania, when she died in a mountain-climbing accident during the summer of 1974.

ALEXANDER LEAF, M.D. (Michigan, 1943), is Internist and Physician-in-Chief, Massachusetts General Hospital and Professor, Harvard Medical School. He has conducted studies in all areas of the world inhabited by supposedly long-lived populations.

ARLENE McCORD, Ph.D. (University of Washington, 1968), is Associate Professor of Sociology, Hunter College, City University of New York. Dr. McCord's major interests are in ethnic minorities, industrial sociology, and education. She is co-author, with William McCord, of *Power and Equity* and *American Social Problems.*

ALAN A. MALINCHAK, M.S. (Florida State University, 1976), Ph.D. candidate (Rutgers University), Assistant Professor of Criminal Justice, St. Thomas Aquinas College, is co-author of *Crime and Criminology* and author of *Criminal Violence and the Elderly.*

CORA MARTIN, Ph.D. (University of Texas, 1965), is Professor and Co-director, Center on Studies of Aging, Texas State University, where she specializes in aging and family relationships.

ZHORES MEDVEDEV, Ph.D. (Agricultural Academy of Moscow, 1950), is Senior Research Scientist in the Genetics Division of the National Institute for Medical Research, London, England. He had worked in medical radiology and genetics until his forced migration from the Soviet Union. He is co-author of *A Question of Madness,* and author of *Molecular–Genetic Mechanism of Development, Soviet Science,* and *Rise and Fall of T. D. Lysenko.*

HUMPHREY OSMOND, M.A. (Guyes Hospital, London, 1942), is Consultant Psychiatrist, Bryce Hospital, Tuscaloosa, Alabama. After serving as a surgeon in World War II, he qualified as a psychiatrist and served at various hospitals in England, Canada, and the United States. His research interests are in psychochemistry, and his published works include co-authorship of *Models of Madness: Models of Medicine and Patienthood: The Rights and Duties of Patients.* He has expertise in socio-architecture of psychiatric hospitals and is, as befits an educated Englishman, a classical scholar.

ERDMAN PALMORE, Ph.D. (Columbia University, 1951), is Professor of Medical Sociology, Duke University. Dr. Palmore is a consultant to the National Council on Aging, the National Institute on Aging (and its predecessors), and to the U.S. Senate Special Committee on Aging. As the references to his work suggest, he is a prolific author and a controversial figure in gerontology.

MATILDA W. RILEY, D.Sc. (Bowdoin College, 1972), is Associate Director for Social and Behavioral Sciences of the National Institute on Aging; Emeritus Professor of Sociology, Rutgers University, and currently on leave from Bowdoin College as Daniel B. Fayerweather Professor of Political Economy and Sociology. She holds, among many distinguished positions, a senior membership on the Institute of Medicine of the National Academy of Sciences. Major publications include *Aging from Birth to Death* and co-authorship of the three volume opus *Aging and Society*.

IRVING ROSOW, Ph.D. (Harvard University, 1955), is Professor of Medical Sociology, Department of Psychiatry and Langley-Porter Neuropsychiatric Institute, University of California, San Francisco. Major works include *Socialization to Old Age* and *Social Integration of the Aged*.

GEORGE SACHER, B.S. (University of Chicago, 1943), beginning his career in the biology of aging with the Metallurgical Laboratory of the University of Chicago (the atom bomb project) and its successor, the Argonne National Laboratories, he was a pioneer in studying the effects of radiological damage to cells and its analogy to the effects of aging. He has been a member of many prestigious groups, including the United Nations Scientific Committee on Effects of Atomic Radiation, and has chaired the advisory Collaborative Committee on Radiology and Health, National Academy of Sciences/National Research Council. He is North American editor of *Experimental Gerontology* and a past president of the Gerontological Society.

K. WARREN SCHAIE, Ph.D. (University of Washington, 1956), is Director, Gerontological Research Institute, Andrus Gerontological Center and Professor of Psychology, University of Southern California. He is editor of *Theory and Methods of Research in Aging* and *Handbook of the Psychology of Aging*.

MIRIAM SIEGLER, M.A. (The New School for Social Research), had her college education interrupted by marriage and childrearing, after which she began training for a career in counseling and psychotherapy. Co-author, with Humphrey Osmond, of "The Dying Role: Its Clinical Importance," she was a consultant at the Anne Sippi Clinic for Schizophrenia in Los Angeles at the time of her death at age fifty.

BERNARD STREHLER, Ph.D. (Johns Hopkins University, 1950), is Section Chief, Gerontology Branch, National Institute on Aging, and prior to that was Director of Aging Research at Baltimore's Veterans' Administration Hospital. His research interests are in aging at the cellular level and mathematical models of age and mortality.

DAN THOMPSON, Ph.D. (University of Chicago, 1972), is Associate Director and Associate Professor of Social Work, Western Michigan University, and previously was planning and evaluation consultant to social welfare agencies in the Midwestern states.

SHELDON TOBIN, Ph.D. (University of Chicago, 1963), is Associate Professor, School of Social Service, University of Chicago. He is author and co-author of many articles and papers and an indefatigable author of review papers in social gerontology.

HAROLD WERSHOW, D.W.S. (University of Pennsylvania, 1960), is Professor of Sociology, University of Alabama in Birmingham. After a career as a social worker with chronically ill and aged, he became a teacher and researcher with a special interest in social policy toward the feeble aged. Being a late bloomer, this is his first book.

HAROLD WILENSKY, Ph.D. (1955), is Professor of Sociology and Research Sociologist in the Institutes of Industrial Relations and International Studies, University of California, Berkeley. Author of several books, including *The Welfare State and Equality*, he is editor of *The Uses of Sociology*.

DOUGLAS WRIGHT, B.A. (Wake Forest University, 1974), is editor and part-owner of *Out* magazine, a journal of entertainment/issues catering to the homophilic community of the Washington, D.C. area. He was formerly a public relations officer for the Administration on Aging, DHEW, and an aide to several congressmen.

Part One
Introduction

Introduction

After completing this work, I happened to read Magda Denes's *In Necessity and Sorrow: Life and Death in an Abortion Hospital* (1976). The introduction to her book covered the same themes that are stressed herein and are appropriate to introduce this volume.

> My rage throughout these pages is at the human predicament. At the finitude of our lives, at our nakedness, at the absurdity of our perpetual ambivalence toward the terror of life and toward the horror of death. . . . It is also a book about the intransigent tragedies embedded in being human. . . . This is a document of the evasions, multifaceted, clever, and shameful, by which we all live and die. (p. xvii)

To which one can only add, "Amen."

Why should anyone inflict upon the field of gerontology a new book of readings? The answer is that most anthologies come from the same mold, and this one is, we hope, different. The impetus arose out of picking up yet another "new" anthology and reading for the umpteenth time another article informing us that "Science" will in the next decade or two enable us to live, not merely to exist but to live in health and vigor unto the ninth or tenth decade, perhaps even longer. And then? Further, deponent usually sayeth not; but one would suppose that, if "Science" can bring forth such miracles as Alex Comfort (1969, 1974) or Bernard Strehler (1973) promise us, surely control of more mundane physiological matters as inhibiting atherosclerosis and cancer can easily be arranged. Those of us who are not yet irreversibly down the path of senescence can look forward to collapsing cozily, at an advanced age, into a heap of dust like the wonderful one-horse shay. As evidence, if not definitive proof, there is the inevitable article about one or more of the several Shangri-Las that, even today, beam forth hope from Central Asia and Ecuador (Benet, 1971; Leaf, 1973a, 1973b). Zhores Medvedev's (1974) pointed, definitive rejoinder to these dreams is never re-

3

printed, nor are papers that point out the cruel trade-offs necessary for a long life.

We are, after all, products of Western civilization and Americans to boot, that is, the fullest efflorescence of Western civilization. We are all boy scouts; we have only once had a devastating war fought on our own soil, and we really don't accept that tragedy and death are an inevitable part of life (Lerner, 1957).

This then, is an "un-American" reader in gerontology. It will show the other side, the dark, tragic side of life. Medvedev (1974) and Sacher (1977) will be in it. We will raise other disturbing questions, for example, of the concatenation of world crises raised by Rosow (1975), Wershow (1977a, 1979), Club of Rome (1972), and doubtless others, and of the impossibility of providing more and more of better and better services to the aged in competition with needs of other groups in an economy that will certainly not grow as rapidly and may even retrogress in the coming years. We must discuss the distasteful problem of setting priorities in the unending expansion of need for health and welfare services to all age groups. We must also raise the question of why all our brave efforts at social engineering go awry. We have created a public welfare system that in the 1930s would have seemed paradisiacal, but that has swelled into a self-defeating, if not always self-serving, monstrosity. We have, with the very best of intentions, spawned other monsters in public housing, juvenile justice, deinstitutionalization of aged and mental patients. Whatever we do turns not to gold, but to ashes (E. Cohen, 1978).

We plan to put opposing positions side by side, to show how limited is our knowledge of humans and their works. Indeed, how can our knowledge of our own complexity be other than limited, when even our knowledge of physics dissolves into such puzzles as dark holes, quarks, and antimatter, far beyond older paradoxes of light acting now as particles, but then again as waves? Truly, the world is not only more complex than we have imagined. It is probably more complex than we can possibly imagine, and if this is so in physics, how much more complex must human life be?

It is difficult for a scientist to retain the objectivity appropriate to a scientific discipline in a world in which science has left the ivory tower. There was a time when nothing that we did mattered very much. Today, findings, even opinions, of behavioral as well as "hard data" scientists, matter very much. The Bomb brought the physical scientists into public purview; the expansion of research money and the foundation of the National Institutes of Health pushed the natural scientists forward. The awareness of problems of poverty, human aggression, mastering complex organizations, and finding ways of inducing people to submit to, or participate in, activities ranging from immunization drives to the "battles for the hearts and minds of men" have given the behavioral scientists their share of the limelight. The public knows very little about the differences between science and Scientology, astronomy and astrology, chiropractic and medicine, much less about scientific method and the subtleties of experimental and control groups. An ignorant public, and the government it chooses, cannot wisely legislate and administer our science programs, especially in areas dealing with human finitude, suffering, and death. Public and scientists alike run away from the unpleasant visions, the hard decisions, the unyielding facts.

Lewis Lapham (1978) put it well:

> The more that one is reminded of one's mortality, the more this must be denied; the more complicated and threatening the world becomes, the more that people must insist that it is simple. Thus the general retreat into caves of superstition and the closets of fantasy. To wandering saints and evangelicals the faithful pay higher prices than they pay for foreign oil. They take up jogging and hope that if they run far enough and fast enough they will outdistance the black hound, death. (p. 14)

We do not advocate nihilism, though there are areas where the rule "first of all, do no harm" may dictate no more than demonstration and development work until we can do better than we now know how to do. It is our intention to dispute vacuous optimism, to insist on as hard facts as are available, to question facile solutions, to raise embarrassing questions, to tread on established toes. We hope that others will join us, will suggest additional papers to adorn future editions of this work, will argue back at us and remove some of the simpleminded "do good, keep smiling, and hope for the best" attitude that demeans the field of gerontology.

Most readers seem to follow a pattern. After the ritual promises of biological miracles, they sketch out the demographic, economic, and social parameters of the aged, usually limited to the United

States. They may then tell us something about geriatrics, the branch of medicine that deals with diseases of aging. This section, as well as the psychological, social, and economic sections, usually notes in passing, but without much emphasis, the great variability and heterogeneity of the aged. Some have more vitality, more hair, better eyesight, fewer ulcers, and a clearer mind than others half their age. In short, there is great overlap between people of various age groups. After this ritualistic bow, the rest of the reader tells us how terrible it is to be old, how many problems older people have, how poor, decrepit, disabled, senile, isolated, and everything else unfortunate they are. It is most curious that gerontologists (at least those who edit anthologies) seem to be wildly enthusiastic about areas in which the least is known and grasp at straws of hope about which cool heads might display less zeal. They go "ape" over the old charlatans in Shangri-La and about forecasts for the immediate future in molecular biology. Yet genetic engineering is only just past the moment of its conception, and possibilities of intervention in aging "prevention" are no more than speculative. But fields that we know much more about, that present some hopeful aspects, are ignored or only the worst aspects are presented. A large part of the problem of gerontologists, if not gerontology, is that not much is known about nor is much attention paid to the aged who are relatively healthy (85% of the aged are mobile), not poor (about 75% of the aged), nor living alone (almost 70%). This leads to such evaluations of gerontology as Rosow's (1969) critique:

> [U]nfortunately, gerontologists are often myopic and consider the problems they study in a vacuum, as if their disciplines have no light to shed on them. This reflects a commendable involvement with their older subjects, but an unfortunate over-identification with them. For it indicates a crippling vested interest in older "clients" which blinds the investigator. Professional prestige is often subtly affected by the status of the persons one studies. When this is low, as in the case of the aged, professionals tend to deal with the resulting strains in one of two ways. Either they dissociate themselves from their people or else they try to raise their subjects' status artificially, by exhortation. Gerontologists generally take the latter course. For years, they have been intense advocates of the aged at the bar of public opinion. This has come at a profound cost, diverting energy from professional to quasi-political activity, deflecting perspectives from facts to wishful thinking, often compromising the professional

soundness of their work. And the quality of their thinking and research has indeed suffered. Many have all but ignored their own
disciplines and the knowledge about human behavior and social
systems which has been accumulated. The fruits of their commitment to social action have become painfully clear. For the common
parochialism of gerontologists has levied a price on sociology and
psychology as disciplines, on gerontology as a speciality within them,
and in the last analysis on the nation's older people, who might
presumably benefit from our deeper understanding of the forces that
govern their lives. . . . It is time now to engage the problems as social
scientists, with a clear, hard look at the issues and without wishful
thinking or distortion because of our ideological stake in the results.
(p. 257)

Scientific work is not easy. As Arnold Penzias (1979), cowinner
of the Nobel Prize in Physics for 1978, put it:

A scientist has to do two contradictory things. One: Maintain
enthusiasm and interest in your work. Two: Don't care too much, or
you are going to come up with the wrong answer. That is, a scientist
must maintain objectivity. If he doesn't, if he lets his speculations—
the prediction of the answer—get too far ahead of his experiments,
they will turn out to be wish fulfillments. There are too many examples of incorrect experiments because people were convinced what
the answer ought to be. (p. 27)

Readers will find herein a number of examples of loss of scientific objectivity and the influence of ideology in gerontology.

To guide less knowledgeable readers in evaluating their reading and thinking about gerontology, the following "rules" are suggested.

Wershow's "Rules" of Thinking about Gerontology

1. If the findings of a study agree with one's own desires and
beliefs, the evidence for that study should be scrutinized with all the
critical acumen that can be mustered. If the findings are displeasing,
we will, without urging, be sufficiently critical.

2. The Principle of Ockham's Razor (Russell, 1945) is applicable to the social sciences and gerontology. That is, in choosing

between two hypotheses, the one that requires fewer assumptions is more likely to be true.

3. Good studies have properly selected control groups. Where circumstances permit, the design should be double-blinded. If a control group is lacking, be very skeptical of the findings.

4. Poor is worse; old is worse. But the human species often has unimagined strengths. Therefore, neither poverty nor old age may be as bad for everyone as we might imagine them to be.

5. We project our own values, expectations, and beliefs upon other people, who may not share those values. A prime example is the desire to work at a paid job. Given even a barely adequate income, many people, young as well as old, would cheerfully eschew the delights of self-actualization and fulfillment not found in the routine, boring, physically and/or mentally exhausting, and trivial work that most of the human species is forced to endure. But university researchers and teachers, whose work is usually fun and fulfilling, cannot see that.

Some of the articles chosen for this reader and some of our comments may sound impatient, caustic, and/or angry. These feelings grow out of love, not hate: love for the disciplined mind; love for those who attempt to find ways of building responsive institutions (a topic about which we know very little and few dare to contemplate); love for honest thinkers and workers in the vineyards of gerontology, who jump not at conclusions, however wistfully we may wish to believe them. It is these to whom we are humbly grateful for the papers contributed. And to the readers who attempt to choose between degrees of truth and error, of wisdom and foolishness (and who love gerontology enough to attack these questions with some passion), this anthology is humbly (though it may often sound quite opinionated) at their service.

Editor's Note

Some selections have been abridged to eliminate dated information, content irrelevant to the subject at hand, and material repetitive of other presentations. It has also been necessary to shorten some presentations for reasons of space limitations. Every effort has been made to preserve essential arguments and theses. Some material of interest only to specialists and not to the general reader has also been deleted.

In many instances, no more than excerpts from papers have been used; excerpts from some papers are scattered among several chapters. These excerpts are the best replies to the paper that they accompany; they provide succinct alternative viewpoints or contradict other findings. In many instances, the alternative paper, in its entirety, is either not quite relevant and/or too technical for the general reader.

This unconventional format may make it difficult to follow this not-quite-an-anthology and certainly not one individual's creation. Some chapters follow a traditional anthology format—an introduction, several reprinted papers, and a concluding comment by the editor. Others interweave excerpts and portions of papers with other portions of or entire papers of other viewpoints. Please keep this in mind as you read, and you will remain unpuzzled.

1

What Do You Know about Aging?

[This volume] will greatly disturb many people working in aging, not because everything is terrible, but because everything is not so terrible. . . . The image of the elderly that emerged was that of a group of individuals with essentially adequate self-esteem, who were not being destroyed or defeated by anxieties regarding health, crime, or money, who maintained frequent contact with children, grandchildren, and friends, who spend less time watching television or sitting and thinking than the younger interviewers assumed, and who actually saw their lives as better than they had previously anticipated. . . . I wonder with increasing frequency how much we as advocates have become as much a part of the problem as we have part of the solution. (Kalish, 1975, pp. 564–565).

We begin with a short quiz (twenty-five items) that "covers the basic physical, mental and social facts and the most common misconceptions about aging" (Palmore, 1977, p. 315). It is an excellent teaching tool, though it has been criticized because individual items may not correlate well with total scores; seven items (1, 6, 13, 14, 21, 22, 23) may have little utility in differentiating among higher and lower level of information on aging individuals (Klemmack, 1978) and it may not be a good instrument in evaluating bias toward the aged (Holzman and Beck, 1979). Both critics agree that Palmore's quiz is useful in stimulating discussion and thought about aging and in clarifying misconceptions about aging. So, let our readers think, discuss, and overcome their misconceptions. And, if you can forget the simple scoring order, which in our experience as well as Palmore's no one has stumbled upon spontaneously, try it again at the end of the course or after reading this anthology.

Facts on Aging: A Short Quiz

E. Palmore

T   F   1.   The majority of old people (past age 65) are senile (i.e., defective memory, disoriented, or demented).

T   F   2.   All five senses tend to decline in old age.

T   F   3.   Most old people have no interest in, or capacity for, sexual relations.

T   F   4.   Lung capacity tends to decline in old age.

T   F   5.   The majority of old people feel miserable most of the time.

T   F   6.   Physical strength tends to decline in old age.

T   F   7.   At least one-tenth of the aged are living in long-stay institutions (i.e., nursing homes, mental hospitals, homes for the aged, etc.).

T   F   8.   Aged drivers have fewer accidents per person than drivers under age 65.

T   F   9.   Most older workers cannot work as effectively as younger workers.

T   F   10.   About 80% of the aged are healthy enough to carry out their normal activities.

T   F   11.   Most old people are set in their ways and unable to change.

T   F   12.   Old people usually take longer to learn something new.

T   F   13.   It is almost impossible for most old people to learn new things.

T   F   14.   The reaction time of most old people tends to be slower than reaction time of younger people.

T   F   15.   In general, most old people are pretty much alike.

T   F   16.   The majority of old people are seldom bored.

T   F   17.   The majority of old people are socially isolated and lonely.

T   F   18.   Older workers have fewer accidents than younger workers.

T   F   19.   Over 15% of the U.S. population are now age 65 or over.

T   F   20.   Most medical practitioners tend to give low priority to the aged.

T   F   21.   The majority of older people have income below the
                  poverty level (as defined by the Federal Government).

T   F   22.   The majority of old people are working or would like to
                  have some kind of work to do (including housework and
                  volunteer work).

T   F   23.   Older people tend to become more religious as they age.

T   F   24.   The majority of old people are seldom irritated or angry.

T   F   25.   The health and socioeconomic status of older people
                  (compared to younger people) in the year 2000 will
                  probably be about the same as now.

The key to the correct answer is simple: all the odd numbered items
are false and all the even numbered are true. So far, no one taking the quiz
has guessed this pattern of correct answers.

Documentation

(1)   The majority of old people are not senile, that is, defective
memory, disoriented, or demented. Only about 2% or 3% of persons age
65 or over are institutionalized as a result of psychiatric illness (Busse and
Pfeiffer, 1977). A series of eight community surveys found the prevalence
of psychosis (of all types) to range from 4% to 8% (Riley and Foner, 1968).
Thus, all the evidence indicates that there are less than 10% of the aged
who are disoriented or demented. It is more difficult to get accurate
estimates of the proportion with defective memories, partly because of the
different types of memory defects and different methods of measuring it.
However, most studies agree that there is little or no decline with age in
short-term memory storage capacity (using the digit span test). Four
studies did find large age differences in free recall of words, but two of them
found no age differences in recognition of words in a list (Woodruff and
Birren, 1975). As for long-term memory, various community surveys have
found less than 20% of the aged who cannot remember such things as the
past president of the United States, their correct age, birth date, telephone
number, mother's maiden name, address, or the alphabet (Botwinick,
1967; Pfeiffer, 1975). Thus it is clear that the majority of the aged do not
have such serious memory defects.

(2)   All five senses do tend to decline in old age. Most studies agree
that various aspects of vision, hearing, and touch tend to decline in old age.
Some studies of taste and smell have not found a significant decline, but the
best evidence indicates increases in taste and smell thresholds with age
(Riley and Foner, 1968). Studies of structural atrophy in the tongue and

nose with old age support the experimental evidence of decline in taste and smell (Birren, 1959).

(3) The majority of persons past age 65 continue to have both interests in, and capacity for, sexual relations. Masters and Johnson (1966) found that the capacity for satisfying sexual relations continues into the decades of the 70s and 80s for healthy couples. The Duke Longitudinal Studies found that sex continues to play an important role in the lives of most men and the majority of women through the seventh decade of life (Palmore, 1974a).

(4) Lung capacity does tend to decline in old age. Both vital lung capacity (the volume of air that can be forcibly expelled in one breath) and maximum breathing capacity (the volume of air that can be moved in and out of the lungs in fifteen seconds) decline on the average from age 30 onward (Shock, 1962).

(5) The majority of old people do not feel miserable most of the time. Studies of happiness, morale, and life satisfaction either find no significant difference by age groups or find about one-fifth to one-third of the aged score "low" on various happiness or morale scales (Riley and Foner, 1968). A recent national survey found that less than a fourth of persons 65 or over reported that "This is the dreariest time of my life", while a majority said "I am just as happy as when I was younger" (Harris, 1975).

(6) Physical strength does tend to decline in old age. Studies of various kinds of muscular strength show declines in old age compared to young adulthood of 15% to 46% (Birren, 1959).

(7) Only 4.8% of persons 65 or over were residents of any long-stay institutions in 1970 (U.S., Commerce Department, Bureau of the Census, 1970). Even among those age 75 or over, only 9.2% were residents in institutions.

(8) Drivers over age 65 do have fewer accidents per person than drivers under age 65. Older drivers have about the same accident rate per person as middle-aged drivers, but a much lower rate than drivers under age 30 (National Safety Council, 1976). Older drivers tend to drive less miles per year and apparently tend to compensate for any declines in perception and reaction speed by driving more carefully.

(9) The majority of older workers can work as effectively as younger workers. Despite declines in perception and reaction speed under laboratory conditions among the general aged population, studies of older workers (the 12% who are able to continue employment) under actual working conditions generally show that they perform as well as young workers, if not better than younger workers, on most measures. When speed of reaction is important, older workers sometimes produce at lower rates, but

they are at least as accurate and steady in their work as younger workers. Consistency of output tends to increase by age, as older workers perform at steadier rates from week to week than younger workers do. In addition, older workers have less job turnover, less accidents, and less absenteeism than younger workers (Riley and Foner, 1968)

(10)   About 80% of the aged are healthy enough to engage in their normal activities. About 5% of those over age 65 are institutionalized and another 15% among the noninstitutionalized say they are unable to engage in their major activity (such as work or housework) because of chronic conditions. This leaves 80% who are able to engage in their major activity (National Center for Health Statistics, 1974).

(11)   The majority of old people are not "set in their ways and unable to change." There is some evidence that older people tend to become more stable in their attitudes, but it is clear that most older people do change and adapt to the many major events that occur in old age such as retirement, children leaving home, widowhood, moving to new homes, and serious illness. Their political and social attitudes also tend to shift with those of the rest of society, although at a somewhat slower rate than for younger people (Cutler and Kaufman, 1975; Glenn and Hefner, 1972).

(12)   Old people usually take longer to learn something new. Experiments have consistently shown that older people take longer than younger people to learn new material (Botwinick, 1967). Studies of on-the-job trainees also show that older workers tend to take somewhat longer to learn new jobs (Riley and Foner, 1968).

(13)   But it is not impossible for most old people to learn new things. The same studies cited in #12 also show that most older persons can eventually learn new things about as well as younger persons, if given enough time and repetitions of the material to be learned.

(14)   The reaction time of most old people tends to be slower than that of younger people. This is one of the best documented facts about the aged on record. It appears to be true regardless of the kind of reaction that is measured (Botwinick, 1967).

(15)   Most old people are not pretty much alike. There appears to be at least as much difference between older people as there is at any age level; there are the rich and poor, happy and sad, healthy and sick, high and low intelligence, and so on. In fact, some evidence indicates that as people age they tend to become less alike and more heterogeneous on many dimensions (Maddox and Douglas, 1974).

(16)   The majority of old people are seldom bored. Only 17% of persons 65 or over say "not enough to do to keep busy" is a "somewhat serious" or "very serious" problem (Harris, 1975). Another survey found

that two-thirds of the aged said they were never or hardly ever bored (Dean, 1962). The Duke Adaptation Study found that 87% of those 65 or over said they were never bored in the past week.

(17)　The majority of old people are not socially isolated and lonely. About two-thirds of the aged say they are never or hardly ever lonely (Dean, 1962), or say that loneliness is not a serious problem (Harris, 1975). Most older persons have close relatives within easy visiting distance and contacts between them are relatively frequent (Binstock and Shanas, 1976). About half say they "spend a lot of time" socializing with friends (Harris, 1975). About three-fourths of the aged are members of a church or synagogue (Erskine, 1964), and about half attend services at last three times per month (*Catholic Digest*, 1966). Over half belong to other voluntary organizations (Hausknecht, 1962). Thus, between visits with relatives and friends and participation in church and other voluntary organizations, the majority of old people are far from socially isolated.

(18)　Older workers have fewer accidents than younger workers. Most studies agree this is true. For example, a study of 18,000 workers in manufacturing plants found that workers beyond age 65 have about one-half the rate of nondisabling injuries as those under 65, and older workers have substantially lower rates of disabling injuries (Kossoris, 1948).

(19)　Only 10.3% of the population were age 65 or over in 1975 and this will probably not increase to more than 12% by the year 2000, even if completed fertility drops to zero population growth levels (U.S., Commerce Department, Bureau of the Census, 1975).

(20)　Most medical practitioners tend to give low priority to the aged. A series of twelve empirical studies all found that most medical students and doctors, nursing students and nurses, occupational therapy students, psychiatry clinic personnel, and social workers tend to believe the negative stereotypes about the aged and prefer to work with children or younger adults rather than with the aged. Few specialize, or are interested in specializing, in geriatrics (Brown, 1967; Campbell, 1971; Coe, 1967; Cyrus-Lutz and Gaitz, 1972; De Lora and Moses, 1969; Gale and Livesley, 1974; Garfinkel, 1975; Gunter, 1971; Miller, et al., 1976; Mills, 1972; Spence and Geigenbaum, 1968).

(21)　The majority of persons 65 or over have income well above the poverty level. In 1975 there were only 15.3% of the aged below the official poverty level (about $2,400 for an aged individual or $3,000 for an aged couple). Even if the "near poor" are included, the total in or near poverty is only 25.4% (Brotman, 1976).

(22)　Over three-fourths of old people are working or would like to have some kind of work to do (including housework and volunteer work).

There are about 12% of persons 65 or over who are employed, 21% who are retired but say they would like to be employed, 17% who work as housewives, 19% who are not employed but do volunteer work, and another 9% who are not employed and not doing volunteer work but would like to do volunteer work (Harris, 1975). These percentages total to 78%.

(23)   Older people do not tend to become more religious as they age. While it is true that the present generations of older persons tend to be more religious than the younger generations, this appears to be a generational difference (rather than an aging effect) due to the older person's more religious upbringing. In other words, the present older generation has been more religious all their lives rather than becoming more religious as they aged. Longitudinal studies have found no increase in the average religious interest, religious satisfactions, nor religious activities among older people as they age (Blazer and Palmore, 1976).

(24)   The majority of old people are seldom irritated or angry. The Kansas City Study found that over one-half of the aged said they are never or hardly ever irritated, and this proportion increases to two-thirds at age 80 or over. About three-fourths said they are never or hardly ever angry (Dean, 1962). The Duke Adaptation Study found that 90% of persons over age 65 said they were never angry during the past week.

(25)   The health and socioeconomic status of older people (compared to younger people) in the year 2000 will probably be much higher than now. Measures of health, income, occupation, and education among older people are all rising in comparison to those of younger people. By the year 2000, the gaps between older and younger persons in these dimensions will probably be substantially less (Palmore, 1976a).

Part Two
The Biological Dimension

The Biology of Aging

And so, from hour to hour, we ripe and ripe,
And then, from hour to hour, we rot and rot . . .

....

Last scene of all.
That ends this strange eventful history,
Is second childishness and mere oblivion,
Sans teeth, sans eyes, sans taste, sans everything.

Shakespeare, *As You Like It*

Editor's Introduction

So it has been, so it is, and so it will be to the end of time.

This topic is presented first because man is basically a biological being, a product of a long process of evolution of the order primates. It is therefore in this most basic aspect of our being that the problems of gerontology present themselves most clearly and the conflict between "should" and "ought" versus "is" and "can" comes to the fore with utmost clarity. We can hope and wish and fool ourselves, but the finitude of our mortality remains unmoved.

Of course, we have made progress; compare any measures of mortality, morbidity, and longevity in the developed and underdeveloped worlds. We have conquered diseases of childhood to the extent that, except for accidents, very few children die and such rare diseases as leukemia are among major causes of death in children. This is not because so many children die of leukemia, but because so few die of anything else. As one hazard of life is conquered, another must take its place, because the death rate remains one per person; those of us who in earlier ages would have succumbed to dysentery, whooping cough, measles, diptheria, and the litany of what was not so long ago known as "usual infectious diseases of childhood" (UIDC), live to die of heart disease, stroke, cancer, pneumonia, and kidney diseases. And if the present major killers of the aged are conquered, we shall probably live on in the wretched thrall of osteo-arthritis, senility, and other "degenerative diseases of aging," the mirror image of UIDC at the other end of the life cycle.

Whatever we do, however we maneuver, there are trade-offs that probably ensure our current maximum life span. For a long time to come, most of us will die no older than our 70s and 80s. To give an example, there is evidence that ingesting much fewer calories increases the life span of rats. Laboratory rats kept in cages can be semistarved into long life. But no society can keep people in cages merely in order to half-starve them into longevity. Fortunately, this path to longevity won't work in humans. Newer evidence indicates that mortality is higher for low-weight aged than for those who have enough fat on their bones (up to 30% above "ideal" weight) to withstand a seige of illness without becoming emaciated. On the other hand, overweight may encourage hypertension (Butler, 1978). It is equally impractical to live in the torpor induced by a state of hypothermia and to cut down heart disease by substituting polyunsaturated fats for animal fats. Polyunsaturated fats seem to accelerate aging, reduce the effectiveness of immune systems, and increase tumors, again in rats (Pitot, 1977), so doubts arise about human responses to such manipulation.

Some pin their hopes on slowing down the "biological clock" that regulates cell-division and, therefore, longevity. Tampering with the delicate mechanisms of heredity will almost certainly be dangerous. There "ain't no free lunch"; no drug has only one effect (those that do not please us we call "side effects"). Upsetting the balance of a long process of evolution will result in some additional changes in processes that may not be at all welcome. It is wise not to assume any quick cure to growing old. And if one wants to believe that vigorous exercise, prudence in life-styles (no motorcycles, drag-racing, handguns in the glove compartment, no drinking while driving, or better yet no use of alcohol at all) will change the human life span, consider the obstacles. If most hypertensives won't accept a simple regimen of one or two pills several times a day over a long period of time, how on earth will people be persuaded to change entire life-styles? Also, if everybody gives up alcohol, tobacco, steaks, fast driving, stressful challenges, overachievement, and so on, we may live a lot longer. Another possibility is that we will not; it may only seem interminable.

More recent evidence suggests that the problem of altering life-styles may not be as intractable as indicated. Between 1968 and 1975, survival rates of white adults have increased significantly. The chance of survival of the group aged 45 to 65 has increased for males from 27.2 to 28.5 years beyond their current age, an increase of 1.3 years (4.7%)—and from 33.1 to 34.8 years, a 1.6 year increase (4.8%), for females. The group aged 65+ has increased its survival rate proportionately even more—from 12.9 to 13.7 years for males, an increase of 0.8 years (6.2%), and from 16.5 to 18.1 years, an increase of 1.6 years (9.7%) for females. The decrease is due in large part to a decrease in cardiovascular disease of over 20% in that time period (the increase for males aged 75+ was only 10%) (Metropolitan Life Insurance Co., 1979).

These statistics indicate that the educational efforts to control obesity, smoking, and long-term use of antihypertension medication and possibly regular exercise have had more than modest effect. If medical care institutions are able to meet more of the needs of the poor and minorities and as the society makes it possible for them to live by the health-promoting features of the middle-class life-style, we may extend the average life span closer to whatever the biological maximum may be.

Except for the antihypertensive drugs, this victory is not due in large measure to medical progress, but to health education. In the past, medical science has not been the major conqueror of disease. The increase in the life span over the last century has been more the work of the sanitary engineers who separated fresh water from sewage and the advances in living standard than of medicine. Finally, those mythical, long-lived populations are just that—mythical.

Why can't we accept the inevitable? Everything has a price, every problem solved creates a new problem, every disease conquered allows us to die of other diseases, perhaps more drawn out and painful than the earlier ones. Of course, research in basic biological phenomena and clinical medicine must continue; but if the promises are too extravagant, the prospects made to seem too rosy, the payoff delayed too long—the backlash of the irate taxpayer will be as explosive as it has been against the social engineering of the "Great Society," which was oversold, underfunded, and too hurriedly conceived. Advances in our knowledge of basic biology occur over long periods of tedious trial and error, with occasional flashes of serendipity. Clinical advances must become ever slower, complex, and expensive as the easy miracles of infectious diseases are virtually no more. The awesome dilemmas that arise in the application of the enormously expensive technology of treating chronic illness would require a second book. Readers are referred to the irrefutable work of Fuchs (1974) and Knowles (1977).

We summarize here Leaf's (1973a) optimistic view of very old (100 years old and more) yet vigorous people whom he has observed in several exotic areas of the world; following that is a full presentation of Medvedev's (1974) vigorous critique of such views plus an example (Myers, 1978) of how age exaggeration comes about (the example may relate to an almost Revolutionary War veteran, but the way one "becomes" a centenarian is similar worldwide; one is overcome by enthusiasm for notoriety).

Dr. A. Leaf (1973a, 1973b) has investigated several areas whose inhabitants presumably live much longer into a vigorous, healthy old age than do we in modern societies. He visited the best known of these areas—the Andean village of Vilcabamba in Ecuador, Hunza in the Kashmir, which is in the foothills of the Himalaya mountains, and that part of the Soviet Union that lies between the Black and Caspian Seas, which includes the Caucasus, Abkhasia, Armenia, and Georgia.

In Vilcabamba, a Catholic community, baptismal records maintained by the churches supposedly confirmed birth dates, as did testimony from friends, relatives, and neighbors. That one small village, population 819, claims nine centenarians, or 1,100 per 100,000, contrasted with three per 100,000 in the United States. In Hunza, the problem of confirming ages is difficult as their language is unique, has no alphabet, and therefore, no written records. "In some instances, however, the Mir (ruler of Hunza) could, from personal knowledge of his state's history, verify ages," says Leaf. "Yet I had the definite impression of an unusual number of very vigorous old folk clambering over the steep slopes that make up this mountainous land. It was the fitness of many of the elderly rather than their extreme ages that impressed me" (Leaf, 1973a, p. 96). The "best-documented" population of old people exists in the Caucasus. Of greatest credence are baptismal records, but most of the churches have been destroyed, along with their records, and many of the allegedly very aged are not Christians. Weight is also given to passports, letters, and even carvings on door posts and walls that might have recorded important events such as a marriage or birth. Then, too, remembrance of age at marriage, present age of children, and such data were employed as evidence. The reliability of results was checked by asking questions such as these employed with Mrs. Lasuria, who claimed to be 141 years old:

> According to her account, her father lived to be 100 and her mother 101 or 102. She had seven sisters and three brothers, and is the only survivor. Her son, who was born when she was 52, is now 82 (arithmetic: 82 + 52 = 134). She was married the second time at age 50, at the time of the Turkish war—which ended 94 years ago in 1878 (50 + 94 = 144). When she was 20, her first husband almost left home to fight in the Crimean War of 1853–56 (118 + 20 = 138). She started smoking in 1910 when her younger brother died at age 60; he was some ten years younger than she (60 + 10 + 62 = 132). Her second husband, who was two years younger than she, died 28 to 30 years ago, when he was more than 100 (100 + 29 + 2 = 131).
>
> My interview was conducted in such a way that it would have been difficult for each of these assessments to come out in such fair agreement unless a common thread of reality linked them. (Leaf, 1973a, p. 98)

A more skeptical observer might have hypothesized, rather plausibly, that Mrs. Lasuria had been interviewed in the same vein long enough to have gotten a pretty smooth act together and had attained the degree of perfection that delighted those who brought visitors to one of the natural wonders of the Soviet Union.

Leaf's interest extended to the dietary habits of the centenarians of these areas as contributors to longevity. While the Vilcabambans and Hunzans are poor people with much smaller caloric and animal fat intakes than are consumed in affluent societies, the Georgians consume considerably more calories than do most old people, and their intake of milk, yogurt, and cheese (though the cheese is low in fat content) is high. The last group's intake of vodka, and even more, of wine, is considerable. There are overweight, aged Soviet Georgians, a phenomenon Leaf did not believe to be possible. He also learned that all these people exercise vigorously and are also very much honored and full participants in community life. They all also claim sexual potency into unbelievable old age, some women claiming to have given birth to children when they were in their 60s and over. Leaf's writings are replete with delightful descriptions of these extraordinary lively, often wise, and always relaxed old people.

Khafaf Lasuria, the former tea picker, had retired only two years before I met her. When I asked Seliac Butba, aged 121, if he was helping in the construction of a new house springing up next to his own, he responded, "Of course, they can't do without me."

Temur Tarba, a vigorous horse-riding member of the collective farm at Duripshi, had celebrated his hundredth birthday just three weeks before my visit. He showed from his bearing and happy manner that he felt he had "arrived." A few years earlier he had been designated a "Hero of Labor"; he was awarded this high Soviet honor for his cultivation of corn.

He smoked a good deal while I talked to him, but he did not inhale. He devotes the mornings to picking tea and cultivating his garden. "It is best to be a youth," Temur states, "but I have good health, feel well, have wonderful children, and I enjoy myself greatly now." He paused a moment in thought, and then added, "Every day is a gift when you are over a hundred. . . ."

Many of the centenarians emphasized the importance of being independent and free to do the things they enjoyed and wanted to do, and of maintaining a placid state of mind free from worry or emotional strain.

"Now everywhere people don't live so long because they don't live a free life," commented Sonia Kvedzenia of Atara, age 109. "They worry more and don't do what they want." Gabriel Chapnian, 117, of Gulripshi expressed a similar thought when told that few Americans attain his age. His response: "Hmmm . . . too literate!"

Expectation of longevity may also be important. In America the traditional life-span is three score and ten years. But when we asked the young people of Abkhazia how long they expected to live, they generally said, "To a hundred." Dr. Georgi Kaprashvili of Gulripshi confirmed that the public has the notion that the normal life-span of man is 100 years. For exaggeration when proposing toasts, they may say 300 years, but everyone expects to be 100. Are we in the United States perhaps a mortality-ridden society, programming our lives to a shorter existence? (Leaf, 1973a, p. 114)

Editor's Comment

Leaf (n.d.) regrets his enthusiastic and insufficiently critical investigation of the aged of Shangri-La. In reply to our request to use his
paper, he ruefully wrote, "Frankly, I would rather give you permission to burn it," and requested that a statement be added, contain-
ing the newer evidence from Vilcabamba, portions of which follow
herewith.

Statement Regarding the Purported Longevous Peoples of Vilcabamba

A. Leaf

There has long been great interest in individuals and populations which
have attained unusual longevity. Gerontologists are interested in what the
maximal possible human life span would be if all diseases could be stripped
away. Physicians and the public are interested in possible clues which may
indicate how a healthful long life can be achieved.

The Andean village of Vilcabamba in southern Ecuador has received
much attention in the past decade as having an unusual number of very
elderly individuals and an unusual proportion of elders compared with
rural Ecuador generally. . . .

Since the population is of Spanish descent and Catholic, it seemed
that ages should be correct in view of the authenticity which written
Church and civil records should establish. On my first visit in 1970 Miguel
Carpio was pointed out to us by the local authorities and physicians to be
the oldest citizen, aged 121 years. When I returned in 1974, I was startled
to be told that Carpio was then 132 years old! I then asked to see the
baptismal record for Carpio. None could be found. A couple of other
instances, such as that of Micaela Quezada aroused further suspicion about
the correct ages. We were told she was 104 years but careful examination of
the baptismal record provided by the local authorities proved it to be that
of her aunt who bore the same name; the names of the parents on the birth
certificate were indeed different than the names of the parents of the living
Micaela Quezada. Thus, without great care, examination even of existing
records may be quite misleading.

At our workshop on Vilcabamba, held at the Stone House on the NIH campus sponsored jointly by the Fogarty International Center and the National Institute of Aging, most of the individuals who had conducted studies on Vilcabamba were present. . . . At this meeting, Dr. Mazess reported on his study of the Church and civil records to establish the correct ages of the elder citizens of Vilcabamba. He found no living centenarians and the ages of villagers alleged to be centenarians were at a maximum in the mid 90s. He postulated that over the past one or two decades the oldest citizens may have died off.

Professors Mazess and Forman (1979), however, studied the population of Vilcabamba and found that if they corrected for the "out-migration" of individuals from Vilcabamba and the "in-migration" of others into Vilcabamba, there was no difference in the distribution of ages of elderly in Vilcabamba as compared with the remainder of rural Ecuador.

Thus, current evidence indicates that there is now nothing unusual about the ages of the villagers of Vilcabamba. Whether unusual longevity had occurred in Vilcabamba in the past can only be a matter now of speculation, but records referring to the good health and longevity of inhabitants of this area go back over 100 years. Studies of heart function among the elders were reported at the workshop which suggest that their cardiovascular function may be unusually well preserved as compared with persons of equal age elsewhere, but this suggestion warrants further careful study.

Editor's Bridging Comment

Zhores Medvedev, noted Soviet dissident and distinguished gerontologist, wrote the following paper soon after his expulsion from the Soviet Union, which disproves the romantic tales. Too bad; we would all welcome the existence of some real Shangri-Las in some remote corners of the world, which could guide us all to a happy and healthy old age.

One not carried away by enthusiasm might wonder why some gerontologists were (and are) so easily fooled (Benet, 1971). Normal scientific skepticism should have warned investigators that the only plausible explanation for this great concentration of extremely old people in this *one* small village, and no other village in that region, is the simple, "Why, they must be lying!"

Leaf learned, the hard way, that the simple, unlettered Indians were most successful in their con game, luring not only scientists, but tourists, a government health center, and a Japanese developer who plans to build a health spa and longevity research center in Vilcabamba (*Time Magazine*, 27 March 1978). Despite the refutation of the legend, some Arabs may soon build a funicular up the hill! The human species loves to be taken in by optimism, however ill-founded.

Caucasus and Altay Longevity: A Biological or Social Problem?

Z. Medvedev

Interest in the study of aging and life-span has increased significantly during the last few years, and this has renewed the old enigma of the maximum possible longevity of human beings. The problem of peaks in human life-span is very important for research programs. If the life-span normally fluctuates around an average level (about 70–80 years), with a progressive decrease in expected life-span with increased age (the picture typical of Europe, North America, and Japan), then the highest level of longevity is about 105 to 110 years. The number of centenarians in the population is normally about 2 or 3 per 100,000; only one person in a million would reach the age of 105 years, and only one in 40 million would live 110 years (one in a country the size of Britain). Such distribution of life-span would support the idea that normal aging is a multi-channel process, its rate depending upon many specific changes in the human organism and many independent control mechanisms.

But the distribution of maximum life-span in some geographically specific areas is different from this kind of fluctuation, and there is statistically a higher proportion of centenarians in the population, with many individuals reaching the exceptional age of 120, 130, or even 150 and 160 years. This phenomenon would indicate that there is a real secret of longevity, and that the life-span can easily be controlled and prolonged by some comparatively simple external factors. This pattern of life-span variations in the human race would favor the theory predicting one or two (or a few) main causes of aging, and one or two aging rate control mechanisms dependent upon external factors. In the last few years, the opinion of many gerontologists started to move from the first concept to the second, and this move was reflected in many articles in the general press connected with reports about new geographical centers of exceptional longevity. Until recently, the unique region of high longevity was usually associated with the Caucasus mountain area, and more specifically with the Republic of Georgia in the USSR. The belief that Georgians have a significantly high proportion of centenarians and enjoy peaks of life-span between 150 and 160 years was regarded rather skeptically by many experts. But some others tried to connect this with the special mountain environment, unique climatic conditions, and with racial and habitual specificity of the Georgian population.

In addition to this almost legendary region of longevity, some others have been described recently, and the search for new geographic areas of increased life-span is now continuing. In the USSR the Institute of Gerontology, Siberian Institute of Cytology and Genetics, and some other scientific units have studied new centers of longevity. In addition to the Georgian area (Abkhazia and Osetia regions), the whole Caucasus and North Caucasus geographical area, with a population of 21,290,400 (1959 census), was reported as an area of great longevity, with 8,890 centenarians (45 per 100,000) and about 500 persons aged between 120 and 170 (Nagorny, Nikitin, and Bulankin, 1963). . . .

In Georgia and Azerbaijan a special medical research unit has been established specially for this research, and the All-Union Research Institute of Gerontology in Kiev also has a special unit for population and medical research, which has made an extensive analysis of the high longevity phenomenon. People of exceptional age (Machmud Eivasov was 163 in 1971, Muslim Shirali died at the age of 168 in 1973) were under close medical observation. In spite of intensive research, however, no scientific explanations have yet been found to account for the peaks of longevity in all these places. The most common approach, which was popular for a long time—the influence of special conditions in mountain areas—proved to be invalid after investigation into details of the geographical distribution of superlongevity. In Yakutia and Altay Plain areas the climate is extremely cold, dry, and continental. Ecuador has a tropical climate. In Caucasus areas, all possible variations of climate can be found: humid and subtropical in Abkhazia (annual rainfall from 1,100 to 2,000 mm.), dry and more continental in central Georgia and Azerbaijan. In large, relatively flat areas of the North Caucasus, the climate is roughly similar to the so called "corn-belt" of the USA. There is no evident correlation between longevity and mountain level; even in Georgia there are some places at sea level with a higher index of longevity than the nearest mountain regions, and the distribution of this index between mountain populations at equal altitudes is very wide, ranging from figures minimal for Georgia to some maximum indices (Pizhelauri and Lugovoi, 1962). About 23% of Georgian territory is between sea level and five hundred meters above.

Factors of genetic inheritance, which might provide possible explanation for isolated villages cannot be used either for the Caucasus or Altay areas. Both are multinational (more than twenty different nationalities with their own languages in the Caucasus and about ten different groups in Altay). In the past the Caucasus was often conquered (by the Mongols, Turkey, Persia, and finally Russia), and the Altay area was also conquered by its neighbors. The Caucasian nations actively participated in trade travels between Europe and the East, and among Altay nationals marriages between tribal relatives were forbidden. Berdyshev (1966) proposed that the multinational character of these centers of longevity suggest the possible role of genetic hybridization (heterosis), but there is no real evidence that the level of mixed marriages here is higher than in other multinational areas of the world. Living conditions are also very complex and different. If the restricted consumption of calories in Ecuador and Hunza is considered, then the Georgian and Caucasus nationals have had very high standards of nutrition for centuries, and the consumption of wine in Georgia is traditionally very high, probably higher than in France.

My own interest in the problem of exceptional longevity in the Caucasus area began long ago when I was a young student at secondary school and lived in Tbilisi, and capital of Georgia, from 1941 to 1942. I was already interested in biology and the problem of aging and was fascinated by the reports published by Bogomoletz (1940) and his colleagues about the first scientific expedition to Georgia in 1937 (organized by the Liev Institute of Clinical Physiology) to study the physiological and health conditions of the large group of centenarians in the Abkhasian part of Georgia. . . .

But after collecting and analyzing information about this remarkable longevity in many areas of the USSR, I nevertheless came to the following conclusion. In most cases the phenomenon of exceptional longevity restricted by specific geographical areas does not exist, and a lot of direct and indirect information strongly suggests that we have in this neither a medical nor biological problem, but a complex social problem which developed for many social, cultural, habitual, traditional, local, and political reasons and which was backed by science under conditions which normally lead to the transformation of science into pseudoscience, conditions which do not permit real objective and neutral or critical study, and which intentionally produce only conforming information.

Listed below are the main factors and conditions which are responsible for the high longevity puzzle in some areas of the USSR.

(1) State statistical documents about age distribution in the population of the USSR based on the periodical All-Union Censuses cannot be valid for scientific research, especially in the oldest groups, because all informa-

tion collected in census questionnaires is prepared from verbal answers without presentation of documents. The doubtfulness of information about centenarians is clear from a comparison of the results of the censuses of 1926, 1959, and 1970. The general census of 1926 estimated 29,000 persons over the age of 100 in the USSR, when the total population was 170,000,000 and average life-span 42 years. In 1959 the average life-span was 67 years and total population about 240,000,000, but the number of centenarians decreased to 21,000. This means that the number of centenarians per million had decreased about two times. The census of 1970 registered a further drop in the total number of centenarians in the USSR to 19,304. However, in the Caucasus area during the same period, between 1926 and 1959, the number of centenarians increased, and the whole "high longevity phenomenon" was localized chiefly in the Caucasus, especially for persons older than 120 years (but the census of 1970 also showed a decrease in the number of centenarians in the Caucasus from 8,890 to 4,925). This change in distribution pattern of high longevity is most probably connected with the fact that the significant improvement in cultural and educational level of the population of Russia reduced the possibility of collecting wrong or false information. The same thing happened some time ago in the USA, where the census revealed many more centenarians among the black population than the white. Black centenarians, of course, had no birth certificates.

(2) Internal passports (or other identity cards) cannot be considered as valid documents confirming the age of old persons in the USSR, because the existing passport system was introduced only in 1932, and is in use for the urban population only. In 1932 dates of birth were inserted in passports from oral information only, without birth certificates. The country population has no passport system up to now.

(3) In Moslem areas of the Caucasus (Azerbaijan, Abkhasia, Dagestan, Adzaria, and others), where the proportion of centenarians is greatest, there was no birth registration at all. There was no birth registration in the Altay and Yakut areas of Siberia. In Christian areas of Caucasus (most of Georgia, Armenia), birth registrations before 1917 were made in the special local church registers, but this registration was not connected with the preparation of special birth certificates. Since about 90% of all churches were destroyed between 1922 and 1940, it is practically impossible to study these church registers now.

(4) Not one of 500 famous long-lived persons claiming to be between 120 and 170 years old was able to produce reliable documents about birth, education, military service, date of marriage, etc., and all reports of research expeditions were based on indirect interviews with relatives,

memories about past events, etc. This situation is also usual for many centenarians in these areas claiming an age of 100 to 120.

(5) Areas of the Caucasus with a high and old Christian culture (Armenia and some parts of Georgia), which voluntarily joined Russia about 400 years ago, have a significantly lower porportion of centenarians than Moslem areas which were conquered by Russia as a result of the long war which lasted several decades in the 19th century. It is also possible that the Moslem year, which has a 10-month duration, caused some misunderstanding when these nationals faced the registration of their ages.

(6) In the Altay area of high longevity, the number of centenarians is three to four times higher among many local Altay nationals (mixture of Mongolian and East European races) than among Russians living there since the seventeenth century, having higher cultural and living standards and a higher than average life-span. Native Altay nationals, who represent about 30% of the total Altay population, are very heterogenous and include many different tribes (Tabalers, Kumadjins, Chelkanzes, Shorzes, Altay-Kizhis, Telngites, Teleses, and others). They do not have any birth documents, and the age of their centenarians was collected by research expeditions mainly by interviews with other villagers and questions about recall of significant events from the past. The dates of birth in this area, as well as in other areas of the Soviet Middle East, are not registered, but connected with one or other significant event in the history of the local tribe. "I was born during a great famine in our place" or "I was born when famous black hunter died under snowfall"—these are typical replies concerning date of birth (Berdyshev, 1966).

(7) The censuses sometimes revealed higher figures in an older group of centenarians than a younger one or the delay in mortality rate after 100 years of age. In the Altay region, the census of 1959 revealed 15 individuals aged between 111 and 113 years and 19 individuals aged between 114 and 116 years (Berdyshev, 1968). In one district of Dagestan the distribution of centenarians indicated significant delay in mortality rate after 110 years: 72 persons 100 to 104 years old, 44 persons 105 to 109 years old (mortality is 39%), and 39 persons 110 to 114 years old (mortality is 12% in comparison with the previous group) (Alikishiev, 1962). Theoretically such a pattern of age distribution is not possible.

(8) According to general statistics, females have a longer average life-span than men. In the USSR, the ratio of women to men aged between 90 and 99 is about three:one in favor of women. But after 100 years of age, this ratio starts to change in favor of men. In the above-mentioned district of Dagestan there were fifty women and twenty-two men in the 100- to 104-year-old group; twenty-six women and twenty-two men in the 105- to

109-year-old group; seven women and ten men in the 115- to 119-year-old group, and two women and four men in the 130- to 139-year-old group (Alikishiev, 1962). In all the USSR, according to the census of 1959, there were 13,306 women and 4,227 men in the group 100 to 109 years old (74% women); there were 368 women and 224 men in the group of people older than 120 years. But almost all persons older than 150 years were men. It is possible to suggest that men are more likely to try to exaggerate their real age than are women.

(9) There were many reports about simultaneous exceptional longevity of married couples: a Misabecian couple—husband 140 years old, wife 116 years old (their youngest son was born when he was 107 and she was 83 years old) (Nagorny, et al., 1963). Long-lived Ukrainian Pavel Tkachenko, who was 120 years old, reported that his father died at the age of 121 and his mother at the age of 117. His grandfather lived 113 years and his grandmother 126 years (Spaskukozki, et al., 1963). The importance of marriage status for longevity was known, but not to such an extraordinary level.

(10) According to the census of 1959, the average life-span in the Caucasus area is about the same as for the whole Soviet Union. The proportion of old people age between 60 and 70 is also the same. But the number of persons who reach the age of 80 is 40% higher than average, the number of persons who reach the age of 100 is 410% higher, and the proportion of people who reach the age of 110 years is 2,000% higher. If we compare the life expectancy in the Caucasus area with Estonia (Baltic sea area), which has the highest living standards in the USSR, it would be found that the life expectancy in Estonia is higher in the 10-, 20-, 30-, 40-, 50-, and 60-year-old groups, but after 90 years of age the situation changes. In Estonia 1,600 persons per 100,000 reach the age of 80, in Georgia only 1,500. But only two in 1,600 in Estonia reach the age of 100, in comparison with 80 to 90 centenarians in Georgia per 1,500 aged 80 years. In the Altay area only 800 persons in 100,000 reach the age of 80, but the proportion of centenarians is about the same as in Georgia. This indicates that high longevity in Georgia and Altay is not usual for the whole population, but is a certain quality of some special people.

(11) In case reports of research expeditions to the Caucasus and Altay areas, there is a lot of information about falsification of real age and many cases of wrong birth dates in passports. "We met many old persons" Berdyshev, head of the Altay expedition, indicates "who produced oral statements or passports where their age was 150 to 180 years old. But detailed analysis of their family backgrounds and other data proved an arbitrary exaggeration of their real age, sometimes by about two or three times" (Berdyshev, 1966). There were a lot of similar descriptions in the

reports of the Caucasus expeditions, and some persons in Georgia and Azerbaijans claimed to be more than 200 years old.

(12) The distribution of centenarians in Altay and the Caucasus is not random, and usually one village has one centenarian. There are no intellectual or church men with public records or past activity among persons older than 108 years.

(13) Physiological and biochemical studies of Caucasus centenarians do not usually produce the correlations between their age and the level of functional and biochemical changes which is expected. Summarizing many reports at the recent special conference on the centenarians, Frolkis (1973) states, "Study of the health of longevous people usually results in an important paradox. The function and metabolism of longevous people of 100–110 years are on the same level as is usual for people of 55–60 years." Research in other countries concerning centenarians with well-established ages does not usually give such paradoxical results.

Biological or Social Problem?

The only scientific hypothesis about the highly increased proportion of centenarians in some special areas of the USSR has been offered by Berdyshev (1966) who suggested that this may be the result of tribal, racial, or national hybridization (heterosis), and therefore places of high longevity are situated in areas with a mixture of different races and nations. Such a possibility can indeed be considered. However, the real hybridization index between Georgians, Armenians, Azerbaijans, and other nations in the Caucasus and in Altay is not very high, and most mountain villages here are rather isolated. Urban populations where cases of international marriages are most usual have comparatively very few centenarians. High longevity figures in border regions between nations are no different from internal regions.

But there are some important social factors and political situations which must be very seriously considered in any attempt to find a solution to this longevity puzzle and which nobody has yet discussed objectively. I will try to indicate some of them.

(a) The traditional cult of longevity and old age. Berdyshev (1968), who studied the longevity phenomenon in the South Altay area, stated that "In the mountains of South Altay very old people have the highest authority; other villagers visit them to get advice and help in the solution of different problems." This custom is also traditional for Caucasus nationals; the older the person is, the more respect and honor he (or she) receives. Centenarians are usually chairmen of local celebrations, dinners, marriages, etc. The most elderly people are almost regarded as saints. Such traditions create the stimulus to exaggerate age, especially when no documents can prove the real age and there are no living witnesses to remember when the oldest person in the village was really born.

Local honor and publicity surrounding centenarians has been supplemented during recent decades by publicity at district, regional, republican, or even All-Union levels, by articles and pictures in newspapers and magazines, by interviews, by special medical attention, etc. All this induced some kind of competition among villages and districts, and while improved statistics and study of existing records permanently decrease the total number of centenarians per million for the whole country, longevity records are climbing all the time: if 35 years ago these records were about 115 to 120, during the 1940's they reached 130 to 140, and now several persons are considered to be as old as 160 to 170 years.

(b) State propaganda about longevity. In spite of the fact that the general censuses collecting oral information about the age of the population are not valid for the oldest group (because of unreliable memories), the state program of political propaganda frequently refers to the record number of centenarians in the USSR and considers it to be a special social achievement of the Soviet Union. Articles in central newspapers and magazines entitled "The USSR—State of Longevity" (especially ambitious in Georgia, Dagestan, and other local press) create an atmosphere which stimulates the legends and superficial approach instead of serious critical analysis. Even in academic books on aging written by serious gerontologists, it is possible to find statements like "The Soviet Union is the country with the record longevity of human beings. The number of centenarians is increasing parallel with our approach to the creation of a communist society." In 1956 the Ministry of Post and Communication issued a special postage stamp with a picture and congratulation to the oldest citizen in the USSR, Machmud Eivasov (Dagestan), who reached the age of 148 years and was still working on a collective farm. After this, Machmud Eivasov became a kind of national hero, and when I left for Britain more than a year ago he was still alive and approaching the age of 164. But it was recently found that he was not the oldest person in Dagestan, and a picture of his competitor, Muslim Shirali, happily listening to a transistor radio at the age of 167 years was distributed by the Soviet press agency Novosty all over the world. Novosty Press constantly sells abroad pictures and stories about especially long-lived people. In Georgia a special Song and Dance Company was created consisting of about fifty people older than 100 years; this remarkable group is touring Georgia and elsewhere singing and dancing as a vivid advertisement of the outstanding longevity and vitality of centenarians in this proud nation.

(c) *Long live Comrade Stalin!* The most curious aspect of the past anxiety about longevity in Georgia was the fact that Stalin was Georgian (his real name was Dzugashvili). With approaching old age he became very interested in the legends that Georgians can usually live to the age of 100 years. He liked to listen to stories about longevity in Georgia and, of course, local authorities in Georgia tried their best to find more and more cases to prove this belief. The old legend about women from Gorni (the village of Stalin's birth) who died at the age of 180 was considered seriously in some academic books on aging. In the post-war period, when Stalin was about 70 and rumors of his poor health started to circulate, official propagandists and political lecturers usually referred to the Georgian high longevity phenomenon to convince people about the possibilities of long life for the Dear Wise Teacher. Neither Stalin nor Beria liked Armenians, neighbors of Georgia and Azerbaijan, with an ancient Christian culture and high standard of living. It is, therefore, interesting to note that Armenia has the highest average life-span expectancy in the Caucasus area—but only about 200 centenarians per 5,000,000 of its population, or four per 100,000, approximately the level usual for European countries. Probably the increase is connected with the Georgians and Azerbaijans who live in Armenia (about 15% of Armenian population).

(d) *Other social factors.* The famous man from Yakutia, who was found during the 1959 census to be 130 years old, received especially great publicity because he lived in the place with the most terrible climate. (This place is sometimes called the Pole of Cold, because the winter temperature here is –50 C. to –60 C.) When publicity about him became all-national and a large article with a picture of this outstanding man was published in the central government newspaper, *Isvestia*, the puzzle was quickly solved. A letter was received from a group of Ukrainian villagers who recognized this centenarian as a fellow villager who deserted from the army during the First World War and forged documents or used his father's (most usual method of falsification) to escape remobilization. It was found that this man was really only 78 years old. How many other cases like this were possible nobody knows, but it is clear that the number of deserters from the army during the First and Second World Wars and during the Civil War ran into hundreds of thousands. Under such circumstances the increased proportion of centenarians in some places will strike us many years from now. . . .

Editor's Comment

Another example of the politicization of science in the Soviet Union
is the following:

> Professor Grigory Pizhelauri, a Georgian gerontologist, express-
> ed this sentiment in "People of High Longevity in the Central Asian
> Republic of Georgia": "We, the Soviet people, are not frightened by
> the problem of 'aging' of the population which so excites the rulers in
> the capitalist countries where old age is the saddest and most burden-
> some period of life." Labor is considered to be the source of longev-
> ity, and intellectual work is said to strengthen cerebral activity in
> later life. The role of heredity is minimized, and major emphasis is
> placed on the socioeconomic aspects of life. The Russians see the keys
> to a long life as being self-restraint, self-control, and knowing how to
> suppress negative emotions. (Butler, 1978, p. 6)

What better way to survive in a totalitarian society? Many
people with those virtues did not, but mighty few without them did,
survive the Stalinist purges. Self-restraint, self-control, and suppression of negative emotions are useful attributes in any authoritar-
ian system.

The following account shows how old people become very old
and then remarkably old. Old age, like poverty, may be no disgrace,
but in our time it is no great honor either. But to achieve remarkably
old age brings at least notoriety, if not honor.

A small cemetery near Warrior's Mark, Pennsylvania contains
the remains of one Christopher Vanpool, who supposedly died on
October 3, 1866, at the ripe age of 112 years and some months
(Myers, 1978). Several accounts of Mr. Vanpool's life have appeared
in local historical society journals, according to which his birth took
place in Bucks County on May 23, 1754. Though he was 22-years-old
at the time, he did not fight in the Revolutionary War, but he had
allegedly often visited Philadelphia and had seen George Washington and Lafayette as well as General Howe and his redcoats. Mr.
Vanpool lived on a farm near Stormstown, where he worked as a
farmer and tanner from about 1805 until his death.

Since he had lived in one small community for over sixty years,
it was possible to locate his records in five of the six decennial

censuses from 1810 to 1860. His age is accurately reported up until the census of 1850, and these reports are consistent with a birth date of circa 1773, not 1754 (which would have been necessary for him to have been 112 at his death). Between the censuses of 1850 and 1860, Mr. Vanpool aged twenty-seven years (!); he crowded in another eight years between 1860 and his death six years later. He evidently began exaggerating his age in his 80s and was likely to have died at the ripe age of 93 or thereabouts, but hardly 112.

Such is the fate and reputation of centenarians, when hard-nosed scientists investigate their ages. Sic transit gloria mundi!

Recommended Readings

Bunker, J.; Barnes, B.; and Moesteller, F., eds. *Costs, Risks, and Benefits of Surgery*. London: Oxford University Press, 1977.

Fuchs, V. *Who Shall Live: Health, Economics and Social Choice*. New York: Basic Books, 1974.

Knowles, J. *Doing Better and Feeling Worse: Health in the United States*. New York: Norton, 1977.

3

What Are the Possibilities of Extending the Human Life Span beyond Its Present Absolute Maximum of 95–105 Years?

The manner in which animals learn has been much studied in recent years, with a great deal of patient observation and experiment. . . . One may say broadly that all the animals that have been carefully observed have behaved so as to confirm the philosophy in which the observer believed before his observations began. Nay, more, they have all displayed the national characteristics of the observer. Animals studied by Americans rush about frantically, with an incredible display of hustle and pep, and at last achieve the desired result by chance. Animals observed by Germans sit still and think, and at last evolve the solution out of their inner consciousness. To the plain man, such as the present writer, this situation is discouraging. I observe, however, that the type of problem which a man naturally sets to an animal depends upon his own philosophy, and that this probably accounts for the differences in the results.

Bertrand Russell, *Philosophy*

Editor's Introduction

This chapter contains an exposition of the optimistic view of the conquest of the aging process (Strehler, 1973) and some contradictory evidence that is excerpted from various contributions to a symposium on *Extending the Human Life Span* (Neugarten and Havighurst, 1977).

A New Age for Aging

B. Strehler

Growing old is a process that few people care to ponder; indeed, most people skirt the issue by spending a surprising amount of time and effort trying to remain youthful. . . .

We adulate youth and respect age (meaning: I would like to be young again; but there must be something good to look forward to—wisdom, perhaps). We advise friends to stop smoking (meaning: you may be shortening your life). The point is that every human being, whether he admits it or not, is at least vaguely apprehensive about the slow deterioration of his structure and functions that eventually ends in death.

Concern about aging and death is an important component of our subconscious life and may contribute more than is obvious to the increased mental disease among the middle-aged and elderly. Anxiety about the changed role in life that follows the female menopause or vague fears about potency in aging males are stresses that nearly everyone endures in silence despite the reassuring witticism of gerontologist Alex Comfort: "People give up sex for the same reasons they give up bicycling; it looks silly, arthritis makes it painful, or one has no bicycle!"

With all of the deep and hidden concerns about the processes that cause this sense of impermanence, it seems surprising that society has not invested more in trying to understand, control, arrest, or even reverse the underlying causes of aging. On the face of it, nothing would seem more appealing as a goal for the average person than an extension of the healthful years of life. Certainly most men are more curious about the reasons behind their own ephemeral existence on this globe than about the constitution of the rocks on the moon or whether life is present on Mars. But to date, *less has been spent on the entire spectrum of research efforts in biological aging than on a single moon shot. . . .* [italics added—HJW]

Ironically, the same generation that learned to split and harness the atom, cracked the genetic code, and sent men to the moon may be the very one that will *not* benefit from the eventual amelioration of the aging process—a possibility that could become a practical reality before the end of this century. The control of the atom was the product of the urgencies of war; the understanding of how we are specified in long strings of genetic "beads," which each of our cells contains, was the culmination of a century of effort to understand the modes and mechanics of inheritance and gene expression; the conquest of space was prompted by the preceding successes of our competitor's Sputniks. But until now, the conquest of time itself has not been a social objective. . . .

Implicit in the drive for federal support of research in this area is the possibility that men will be able to control—and perhaps reverse—part or all of the aging process. But the only way we can accurately predict what the chances are is to understand the nature of the events that lead to human aging. The transformation of life from a young state to an old one encompasses more than the mere passage of time, but the biological processes involved are not generally understood by the public. Perhaps if the basic principles and the rapidly growing body of new data were more openly discussed there would be greater public support for the needed investment in fundamental research. Only such research, now or in the very near future, may make greatly extended lifetimes available for present generations of humans.

There are two generalizations to keep in mind about the events that occur as we age. The first is that many, although not all, bodily functions decrease gradually as aging takes place. This will not be news to anyone: all schoolboys know they can outrun their grandfathers and that the aged are less active, usually less alert, and more subject to disease than young adults. But this knowledge had not been put on a quantitive basis. During the last thirty years, however, Nathan Shock, the father of American gerontology, and his associates have described the exact rate at which different kinds of bodily functions fail. The essence of these findings is that most functions decrease gradually, at a rate of about one percent of the original capacity per year after age thirty. This means that the reserve ability to do all kinds of work will run out at about age 120. It is not surprising, therefore, that about 118 years is the greatest age attained by any human for whom good records of birth and death are available. . . .

The second generalization is that the *chance of dying does not increase in proportion to the amount of function lost.* [italics added—HJW] This was discovered and formulated into a simple mathematical law in about 1832 by an English insurance actuary, Benjamin Gompertz. *The Gompertz law states that the chance of dying doubles about every eight years, irrespective of the environment in which one lives.* [italics added—HJW] This means that the chance of dying is about 1,000 times greater for a man of 100 than for a man of 25. If we did not age—that is, if we kept the physiology of a 15-year-old indefinitely—the average human life-span would be in excess of 20,000 years. . . .

The basic question, of course, is not do we age, but what is the underlying mechanism. This can be summarized as follows: we age primarily because the cells in our bodies that cannot replace themselves either die or lose a small part of their function every year. This law applies to most of the tissues of the body, although some cells and tissues seem immune to the effects of the passage of time. These non-aging tissues include those covering the surfaces of the body (the skin and the lining of the digestive system) and the circulating cells in our blood. The skin forms a new layer of cells every four days or so, the lining of the gut is replenished every day or two, and the red blood cells are replaced on a regular schedule every four months.

The other body cells, such as those of the liver, replace themselves more slowly, although the liver (of experimental animals) can regrow to its original size within a week or so if part of it is removed surgically. Parts of the kidneys and the connective tissues are able to replace themselves more or less on demand.

Key organs and tissues in which cell replacement is either absent or inadequate are the muscles, heart, brain, and certain endocrine and immunity-conferring tissues. The nonreplenishing, or postmitotic, cells involved exhibit two major differences from those in other parts of the body: many of the cells that remain in the tissues of an old animal are either larger or smaller than usual and the resultant irregular appearance of many old tissues is one of disorder; the second, obvious change is the accumulation of yellow-brown colorations known as age pigments. These materials accumulate slowly with age, and in the very old they may occupy nearly the entire cell body. They are believed to be produced by the reaction of oxygen with unsaturated fats in the membranes within cells. This reaction is similar to the one that causes varnish to harden and turn yellow as it dries and ages.

The rate at which it occurs can be reduced, in the test tube at least, by adding substances call antioxidants to the mixture. In this process the antioxidants trap intermediate molecules, called free radicals, and prevent such reactions from becoming self-perpetuating. Vitamin E is one antioxidant that occurs in nature, and BHT, a synthetic compound used to prevent various food products from turning rancid, has similar effects. One group of studies by Denham Harmon of the University of Nebraska indicates that it is possible to extend the lives of experimental animals by adding antioxidants to their diets. Whether the increased longevity is due to the suppression of antioxidative reactions within cells and tissues is not yet certain.

Recent studies also indicate that cells cultured artificially eventually lose their ability to divide or renew themselves. In his careful and imaginative work in this area, Leonard Hayflick of Stanford University has shown that human cells such as embryonic fibroblasts can only undergo about fifty divisions under artificial conditions. Whether such limitations occur in the body itself is not yet clearly settled. It seems likely that skin and gut cells, for example, are able to divide hundreds or thousands of times during the lifetime of a human. Some recent research suggests that all cells manufacture and accumulate materials that tend to prevent their division when the concentration of these substances is large enough. One class of such substances, called chalones, only inhibits the growth of the tissue from which it is extracted.

Lack of materials that inhibit cell division may contribute to the development of cancer—a disease that primarily affects the elderly. One reason that cancer develops could be that the natural inhibitors, perhaps "chalonelike" substances, are either not produced in adequate amounts or no longer have a growth-stopping effect on cells that have become malignant. This is an oversimplification of the origin of cancer, but several lines of evidence indicate that it is at least a part of the picture.

The key to understanding aging is to be found in the mechanisms that control and prevent the division of cells. Much information may fall out of the understanding of cancer but it seems unlikely that all of the needed facts will result from the pursuit of studies directed toward other goals. What is needed is to focus an adequate research effort specifically on those processes that cause cells to lose vitality with age.

A law of nature states that all systems tend to become more disorganized as time passes unless energy is expended to generate order. Stars burn themselves out; untended gardens go to weed; social institutions become more unmanageable as they age. This also applies to the cells and molecules that make up the individual human being; unless molecules are stored at absolute zero and shielded from all kinds of radiation, they will gradually revert to less ordered arrangements of their atoms.

In one sense, living systems are an exception to this rule, for plants and animals do create order out of chaos. These living organisms are special kinds of machines, which harness the matter and energy about them in order to make more of their kind.

The basic reason that living things are mortal is that this must have favored their evolutionary success. One explanation for this paradox—the death of individuals favoring the perpetuation of the species—was suggested by Peter Medawar, a Nobel laureate in medicine and physiology, who pointed out that some kinds of successful adaptations carry with them side effects that indirectly lead to aging and death. For humans, three such adaptations are particularly important: man is best able to function if he has a particular size; man's brain serves as an information storage device, as well as in other ways; our ancestors evolved in competitive environments, which placed a premium on the efficient use of raw materials. What unites these adaptations is that they all involve the "switching off" of certain inherited abilities at specific times in the life-cycle, and it is this process that ultimately causes the system to fail.

The limitation of the human body to a certain optimum size is achieved by the turning off of the genes that would lead to continued growth. The stabilization of memory elements in the brain is achieved, in part, by suppressing the ability of nerve cells in the brain to divide (nerve cell division is a great rarity after birth). Economy in the use of raw materials requires that only those parts that deteriorate rapidly—the skin, gut lining cells, blood cells—are regularly replaced. Tendons, muscles, heart, and brain cells stop replacing themselves as maturity is approached.

The consequence of this switching off of genes is to remove the affected cells from the "living system" category, as defined earlier, with aging and death eventually following. Yet all cells, whether in a functioning or switched-off state, contain the necessary genetic instructions to replenish themselves. When we discover how to unlock the information hidden in the DNA of each nonreplenishing cell, man may indeed possess the knowledge necessary to convert himself into an immortal.

Before the present revolution in biological thinking—the result of understanding how DNA stores the instructions to put the body's parts together—we had exceedingly cumbersome ideas about the regulation of gene expression. It had been thought that each specific event in each kind of cell was controlled by a huge set of genetic instructions. It seemed inconceivable that man could devise nondestructive means of interfering with the enormous complexity of the regulating systems involved.

But it has now been demonstrated that the genetic code is really very simple. It was proven that it is a sequence of just three consecutive "beads," the nucleotide bases in the DNA, which code for a given kind of building block in the working parts of cells. (The building blocks are the body's total of twenty different kinds of amino acids, and the working parts are proteins, which are simply long chains of amino acids arranged in very specific ways according to the instructions provided by the DNA.)

It also has been shown that only two different types of control locations are involved in the regulation of which kinds of genes are expressed. These sites, on the surfaces of the DNA and of the ribosomes control the copying of the information in specific segments of DNA—a process called transcription—and the decoding of this copied information—a process called translation. In other words, cells can select which of the many products they will make by either controlling the kinds of DNA copied or the kinds of messages decoded.

The importance of these discoveries in terms of the potential control of human aging is enormous. Instead of an imponderable array of control points, the number may be quite small, perhaps only a few dozen. This implies the possibility of producing chemical agents that will selectively change the controls of switched-off cells, thus releasing the latent genetic information needed to produce replacement parts—just as it is possible to produce antibiotics that will destroy infective bacteria without materially harming the body's functions. And far from being an unattainable goal in this generation of humans, selective production of new cells and tissues through pharmacological intervention is on the verge of being tested; at least the basic technology is at hand.

Whether this optimistic view is justified will depend on the results of experiments designed to test a theory of gene regulation proposed about ten years ago. Harvey Itano, now a professor at the University of California at San Diego, suggested that certain genetic diseases are due to the inability of cells to translate some of the code words present in genetic messages. . . .

The basic idea behind the thinking and experiments is that as cells mature they may shut off the ability to read, or decode, certain code words. The effect would be that all genetic messages written down in sequences that include nondecodable words could not be used to produce working parts of cells, including replacement parts.

Editor's Summary

If one might summarize a rather involved description of the genetic code, Strehler tells us that the reproduction of cells is governed by different combinations of "genetic language" that contain at least "one word" for each of the twenty amino acids. Different kinds of cells operate on different combinations of code words, of which there are about sixty. Since there are only twenty amino acids and sixty code words, a protein a hundred amino acids in length (which would be an average simple protein) can be expressed in 3^{100} different ways. There are at least ten thousand different sets of code words, which could specify ten thousand different kinds of cells. The body hasn't anywhere near that many different tissues (that is, groups of the same kind of cell).

If this is true, certain steps needed in translating the instructions carried in the DNA will be accomplished by certain kinds of cells and not by others, a finding substantiated by over fifty different studies. For example, Beck and Strehler have shown that old soybean cotyledon tissue is unable to attach the correct amino acid to the proper decoder molecule, though young tissue does this readily.

Also, old tissue manufactures a substance that blocks the production of materials needed for indefinite existence, but this blockage can be avoided by application of a plant hormone, kinetin, to the tissue while it is young. So some possibility exists of reversing or arresting cell aging. Strehler and Johnson have also learned, using dog tissue, that nondividing cells lose rDNA, which is essential to producing working proteins in the nondividing cells, such as heart, brain and skeletal muscle. The following excerpts from Strehler explore implications of these and other findings.

[L]iver and kidney cells, for example, do not show such losses. The net effect of the gradual loss of some of this genetic material would be to reduce the maximum rate at which protein could be synthesized under stress. Thus, such different afflictions of the elderly as heart failure (which requires the manufacture of heart muscle proteins if it is to be prevented), inability to detect and reject cancer cells (which requires the rapid manufacture of antibody-like substances to kill off the aberrant cells), and a decrease in the efficiency of the hormonal systems (such as occurs in adult-onset diabetes) may all be ascribable to this fundamental loss of rDNA in non-dividing cells. Studies are now under way to test a few of these implications.

It would be too sanguine to state at this time that vital functions could be regenerated simply by reinstating lost abilities to decode one or a few code words. What is needed, of course, is research to find out whether this simple, though versatile, mechanism really dominates the control of development and aging. . . .

Barring unforeseen breakthroughs in other areas of bio-medicine that might provide important insights into the aging process, the key, limiting factor is whether the needed specific effort will be supported by society. This is an unsettled question right now.

One reason that research on aging has not received the emphasis it deserves has to do with the aging of bureaucracies themselves. New bureaus and institutes are often vital organizations; as they grow older they are concerned more with maintaining the status quo than with imaginative progress. . . .

The eventual understanding and control of the aging process will cause a revolution in human affairs. Already a few studies are under way on the social consequences of greatly retarding or abolishing aging and death. A few misconceptions should, however, first be laid to rest. Some of the evidently misinformed opponents of greater, healthy life-spans seem to believe that the world would become populated with decrepit, patched-up, wizened, senile people, perhaps fed through tubes and moving with the aid of electronic prostheses. This ugly picture is totally false, for there is no way to appreciably increase life-span except by improving the body's physical state. Instead, humans that live for 150 years or more will be healthy for a much greater percentage of their total life-span. Men and women of highly advanced age will possess bodies like those of much younger people. In fact, their minds will be even more improved, for the greater years of optimum health will provide more opportunity to assimilate the world's wonders and lead to a greater measure of wisdom—the only intellectual commodity that often improves with age.

Because the healthy middle years of life will be doubled from the present 30 or 40 years, each individual will spend more time as a contributor to society. [italics added—HJW] The average professional of today requires 25 to 30 years to acquire his training—mostly at the expense of the producing members of society. If the post-training years were doubled, every person could give much more back to the pool of resources from which he derived his start.

As the societies of the world evolve, there will be many changes in the kinds of creative activities open to men and women. People with many decades of optimum health will find it desirable, if not necessary, to move from one kind of occupation to another. One way in which continual retraining in new skills and professions could well take place would be through a regular system of educational leaves-with-pay, much like the sabbatical system that now operates in universities. Every five or seven years, a person could take a year or so to acquire new skills and to refurbish old ones. Plans would be made now for the restructuring of educational institutions so that a continuing re-education will become the rule rather than the exception.

As machines take over the more onerous and repetitive tasks men have performed, opportunities for new careers in the so-called service area will evolve. It is unfortunate that there is not a better word than service (from the same root as the word servant) to describe the kinds of creative things people can do to make each other's lives enjoyable. Such efforts range from art, music, poetry, and beautiful gardens, to the care of children, entertainment, and creative conversation. As men escape from a subsistence society, in which work must be done to provide for life's necessities, a much more fulfilling kind of work, one directed toward the improved enjoyment of life, will come to dominate.

In time, all of these joyous prophecies will probably come about anyway, provided we have wisdom, foresight, and a little luck. But they will be available to those who read these pages only if the minuscule investment needed to understand and perhaps control human aging is made in this coming decade. What is commonly termed the Protestant ethic encourages some sacrifice now (work, saving, investment, education, research) in order to derive greater benefits in the future. After nearly a decade of disparagement and eclipse, it seems once again to be revealing its wisdom. One can only hope that this resurgence in the appreciation of investment will extend to what is needed to assure a healthier, longer life for all—basic research on the most universal human affliction, aging itself.

Editor's Comment

Several of Strehler's statements seem to be, at best, questionable, especially the ones italicized on pages 39, 40, and 46. We present here a different viewpoint on these issues.

1. *Strehler's interpretation of Gompertz's Law.*

I cannot understand his interpretation of Gompertz's Law. If the chance of dying doubles every eight years, and physiological functioning does decrease with age (however varied in different tissues), then obviously the chance of dying *does* increase as function is lost. When any one vital system can no longer support life, the person dies, and vitality of many organs does decrease with age, though not *linearly*, but exponentially. The author is technically correct in stating that the "chance of dying does not increase in (linear) proportion to the amount of function lost."

Even if the death rate at older ages, for example, 75+, were to be cut in half, it would add very few older people to the population. If this were to occur, using U.S. 1975 life tables (Vital Health Statistics, 1977), instead of 35,500 white females surviving beyond age 85, 50,000 would live. The life expectancy of that cohort would increase from 6.4 years to 6.75, an increase of less than four months, so powerful is the effect of the high death rate of older people. The current increase in older people is, as was earlier stated, a result of the phenomenal decrease in deaths of younger people. More people survive to die old; the survival of the very aged is not increased substantially and is not likely to change in the forseeable future.

2. *Strehler's call for greater expenditures for basic biological research on aging.*

Goddard's views on the question are presented on page 58–59. We present some points here.

The efficiency of expenditure of funds upon research is directly related to the degree of theoretical understanding of the problems at hand. Once Goddard raised his first primitive rocket some feet off the Arizona desert or Einstein postulated plausibly that $E = Mc^2$, everything else was a matter of technical details. Once we know where we are going, it is not that hard to get there. But until this basic knowledge exists, large expenditures of funds are likely to be merely frustrating. Witness the slow progress in the conquest of chronic disease. The life span increased nineteen years from 1900 to 1952, due to our ability to deal with infectious diseases following development of antibiotics and immunizations against bacterial and viral diseases and even more important, improved sanitation and diet.

Since 1950, the life span has increased less than 2.5 years, because we do not have a handle on the probably multiple paths of causality of rapidly growing parasitic cells of cancer and the clogging up of arteries with cholesterol. Today, most deaths occur in later life. So few die before maturity that, if no one died under age 35, the life span would be extended no more than 3.1 years (Reinhart, personal communication). Dramatic prolongation of life via cures of chronic diseases is illusory. If the work of the National Heart, Lung, and Blood Institute to eradicate cardiovascular disease is successful, it has been estimated that theoretically more than eleven years would be added to the average human life expectancy. This increase is only theoretical because the elimination of one disease would leave people vulnerable to others. The absence of heart disease, for example, might mean that people would die of cancer. A more realistic estimate of the increase in life expectancy as the result of the eradication of heart disease would be four years (Butler, 1978).

3. *On the inadvisability of retirement for older people.*

Strehler has fallen into the same error as has part of the feminist movement. He assumes that most jobs will be skilled, professional, self-actualizing occupations. Unfortunately, even the computer requires more code clerks and key punchers than it does more creative workers. One may even question the creativity of most programming. We may assume that most people will continue to work at boring, routine, meaningless work in the future, as in the past, a point well made by Kalish (1972).

Of Social Values and the Dying: A Defense of Disengagement

R. A. Kalish

A common example of the geriactivistic error is to judge older people by their expressed desire to return to a productive working career. Those who make explicit their enjoyment of retirement are looked at critically, while those who eagerly espouse their inclination to be working are subtly rewarded with approval. The geriactivist is a leader of the let's-get-older-folk-back-to-work movement, always verbalized as a method to enhance the self-esteem of the elderly. That the older person's failures will inevitably increase, that he may be sick and tired of work, that he must eventually leave work anyway, all this is not heeded. Thus the future failure is intensified by placing so much honor upon work and activity. The alternative, equally impractical but at least theoretically preferable, is to enable the older person to understand that his worth as a human being does not depend upon work, that he has earned his right to utilize his time as he pleases in the future, that his forty years of nonactualizing work is not going to be rewarded by permission to pursue another decade of nonactualizing work. . . . (pp. 90–91)

Editor's Bridging Comment: The Case against
Dramatic Breakthroughs in Retarding Aging

Strehler and Comfort are in the minority of gerontological biologists
who believe in the possibility of imminent, that is, before the year
2000 or thereabouts, breakthroughs in the retardation of aging at the
level of cells and tissues. The argument to the contrary presented
here is drawn from the 1977 symposium edited by B. L. Neugarten
and R. L. Havighurst.

Perspectives on Human Longevity

L. Hayflick

Tampering with our Biological Clocks

If the control of aging is dependent upon understanding the basic
biological processes, one profoundly important question arises: How desirable is it to be able to manipulate our biological clocks? The answer to this
question is not simple. The fact that it must be asked is further evidence of
the distinction that must be made between disease-oriented biomedical
research and gerontological research. Who would ask: What are the goals
of cancer research or what are the goals of cardiovascular research? The
answers are so obvious as to preclude asking the question. But the goals of
gerontological research are quite a different matter, because we are not
certain whether the "resolution" of the physiological decrements of old age
will indeed benefit the individual or the society as a whole.

Many different biological resolutions of age changes are possible, and
each has an important potential side effect. Take, for example, the possibility that research into the biology of aging might result in the total elimination of all age-related physiological decrements. . . . [If] this were
achieved, and no control existed on the biological clock itself, the result
would be a society whose members would live full, physically vigorous,
youthful lives until the stroke of midnight on their hundredth birthday—at
which time they would die. If, on the other hand, we were to learn how to
tamper with our biological clocks, with what goal in mind would one choose

to reset his clock? Surely one wouldn't choose to spend an additional ten years suffering from the infirmities of old age—yet that might, initially, be the only way to intervene. Is society prepared to cope with individuals whose only choice might be between naturally occurring death and ten or more years spent with the vicissitudes of old age? We can hardly deal with a mean maximum lifespan of, say eighty years, to say nothing of the further social, economic, and political dislocations that might occur if we add another ten years. . . .

Goals for the Old

. . . In spite of the apparent dilemma in stating goals for gerontological research, one goal appears to be wholly desirable and even attainable as a short-range objective. That is simply to reduce the physiological decrements associated with biological aging so that vigorous, productive, non-dependent life would be led up until the mean maximum lifespan of, say one hundred years. Implicit in this notion is that the quality of life is more important than its quantity. . . .

If longevity is to be increased merely by extending the years of our infirmities, then the goal is not worth seeking. This indeed is the modern dilemma faced by many physicians who are torn between using every means for prolonging the terminal stages of disease in the name of prolonging life but at the expense of continuing the agony of certain death. The goal that is not only more desirable, but indeed more attainable, is not the extension of longevity per se, but the extension of our most vigorous and productive years. If tampering with our biological clocks ever becomes a reality, it would be tragic if such clock tampering would result only in the extension of those years spent in declining physical and mental health. Having said this, what are the prospects of achieving the goal? I believe that the prospects are beginning to brighten.

Changing Attitudes

It is sometimes observed that there are no gerontologists, just biochemists, cell biologists, and immunologists working in gerontology. Many serious biologists with an interest in aging still hold at arm's length the appellation "gerontologist," either because of the attitude that the problem is simply too complex to yield to experimentation, or because the many pseudo-scientific fringe groups in search of biological immortality have had such a pervasive influence that to formally associate oneself with the field is to suffer an unseemly stigma.

Happily in the past few years a significant change in attitude has occurred toward the science of gerontology. There is now the realization that biological aging is no more complex than are problems in embryology, development, neurobiology, cancer research, or genetics. The attitude is untenable that efforts by gerontologists to reverse the aging process are akin to medieval alchemy, for all successful biomedical research has the net effect of prolonging life. Thus there is no rational reason to discourage research on the fundamental causes of age changes. Established investigators are no longer apologetically explaining their interest in aging, and young scientists are beginning to appreciate that the fundamental problems are less intractable than their predecessors thought. Public awareness of this neglected field has led, for one thing, to the creation of an Institute on Aging in the National Institutes of Health.

For the first time the discipline of gerontology has been given a degree of national recognition at the biomedical level, to make real meaningful efforts to understand the biology of aging. The field has now been given a level of national visibility that is almost compatible with the magnitude of the problem. Even more important is the implication that something can and should be done about biological age changes. The period of utter disregard of the question has now passed.

Prognostications

In any attempt at futurology it is wisest to base predictions on similar events that have happened in the past. To the question, What will be the impact of achieving a 5, 10 or even 20-year increase in human life expectancy, we have only to look back at the same question asked in 1900, for it is only during the period 1900–1950 that increases in human longevity of these magntiudes did, indeed, occur. It is therefore safe to conclude that any further increase in human life expectancy is likely to incur the same sets of problems and solutions to those problems that occurred in the first half of this century. The question then is: To prepare for a potential increase in human longevity, what should we now do that is different from what was or was not done in 1900? The chief medical problem during the first half of the twentieth century was infectious disease, and the chief biomedical acomplishment during that time was their virtual elimination. As a result society now finds itself burdened with unprecedented numbers of disabled and indigent old people who have survived infectious diseases but who will not survive old age. We do not wish to prolong old age by keeping people alive well beyond their years of vigor. What we want to do is what the science of gerontology is all about. . . .

Since life expectancy has increased so dramatically in the last half century anyone can forsee the possibility of some small degree of further extension. All that needs to be done is to better the hygienic, health care, and nutritional deficiencies of the substantial proportion of Americans who are now denied these basic human needs. Thus there is no requirement for new intellectual bases of understanding the biology of aging to materially increase the longevity of a substantial portion of our society. All that it takes is motivation and money. This achievement would increase life expectation but, of course, would not affect the lifespan or the rate of aging. Nevertheless, it is something that could be done now without requiring any new scientific innovations.

For significant increases in longevity to take place, spectacular scientific achievements will be necessary.

The consensus of scientific opinion is that the fundamental causes of age changes, like developmental changes, are somehow programmed within the genetic apparatus. It is there that the clock is undoubtedly located. A fruit fly is old in thirty days, a mouse in three years, and a man in ninety years. The genetic control of these differences is more or less self-evident. The rate of aging per gram of mouse tissue is thirty times faster than per gram of human tissue. Further clues that genetic processes control age changes can be seen from the sex differences in human and animal life expectation. Perhaps the best examples are actuarial data which clearly show that the children of long-lived parents are themselves long-lived. Demographic data lead to the amusing conclusion that the best possible circumstances for achieving maximum longevity are to be a white, highly educated, wealthy, Swedish female with centenarian parents and grandparents (one wonders what such women would have to say to her poor old, black, sick counterpart living in an American ghetto).

The conclusion to be reached, then, is that if, in the next twenty-five years, biomedical research were to triumph to the extent that deaths caused by cardiovascular disease and cancer would be preventable, a net increase in life expectancy of about twenty years* would occur. Advances made in preventing deaths caused by other diseases would not have much impact on human longevity. The greatest potential impact on human longevity would be research directed toward reducing the rate of the fundamental non-disease-related biological causes of age changes, causes which are undoubtedly genetically determined.

If our social, political, and economic institutions are likely to be severely dislocated by these achievements, what right do we have to encourage this kind of research? (pp. 10–12).

---

*Hayflick now estimates the increase in life expectancy at fourteen years (personal communication, 1980).

Editor's Bridging Comment

Havighurst and Sacher (1977) continue the discussion of the un-
likelihood of extending the life span. We can help more people to
live to be old, but are unlikely to find ways to enable a larger
proportion of the people to live to be very old.

Prospects of Lengthening Life and Vigor

R. Havighurst and G. Sacher

Two Ways Of Extending The Mean Lifespan

(1) Slowing the rate of aging. . . . Thus far no pharmacological
method has been demonstrated that slows down the rate of aging, even in
smaller animals. Several "antiaging" drugs or chemicals that have been
used with mice and other small animals have prolonged the lives of these
animals. . . . The "antiaging" substances extend lives by helping the
animals resist the ordinary diseases which cause death, but *these antiaging
substances do not greatly extend the maximum lifespan of the animal.*
[Italics added—HJW]
    There are two kinds of regimes that do extend life for experimental
animals by decreasing the rate of aging and that do therefore extend their
maximum lifespans. The first is by restricting the food of rats and mice to
the point of slowing down the animals' activity; the second is by reducing
the body temperature of coldblooded species, insects, and fish.
    How might these methods be applied to humans? It is generally
supposed that most people in affluent societies eat too much, and would be
healthier if they ate less. But this assumption is based on the facts about the
dangers to health of excess fat. Just following a "reasonable" diet will keep a
person's weight down to a healthy normal, but it will not slow the rate of
aging of the cells in the body. To actually reduce the rate of aging of the
cells, it would probably be necessary to reduce the intake of food drastically, or if not the intake itself, at least the body's absorption of nutrients. (The
latter might be accomplished by taking pharmacological substances which
would prevent the body from absorbing nutrients, even though the person
eats all he wants.) The body would not get the nutrition, and would

therefore enter a state of slow starvation. This might slow down the rate of aging of body cells, but it would also slow down the body's activity, for the available energy from food would be reduced, and the person would become listless. The questions would then become: Would people want to pay this price for an extra ten years of existence?

The second method of slowing the rate of aging, reducing body temperature, can be carried out with coldblooded animals like fishes, but can hardly be done with humans. When the human body temperature drops a degree or two below normal, the body starts to shiver, which is a way of making the body exercise itself and thus raise its temperature back to normal. Still, biochemists might discover chemicals that would reduce the temperature of the human body by, say, five degrees, and thereby slow down all body processes, including the processes of aging of cells. But this would make the body less active, and reduce what Sacher refers to as productive energy output. The body would slow down, all mental and physical body processes would slow down. Again, would people want to extend their lives by this method?

(2) *Improving "vigor."* . . .[Some attempts to retard aging are] based on the assumption of a change in the vigor or vulnerability factor. This change can be brought about in two general ways; one way is by improved health practices and health services. Increased vigor and decreased susceptibility to disease have, of course, been going on at all age levels, although very slowly among persons 65+. As mentioned earlier, the use of antibiotics has been one of the ways in which mortality has been greatly reduced; and various public health measures have had the same effect. For present purposes, however, we are speaking of health practices that might begin at age 40, when, for example, reduction of cigarette smoking, maintenance of low cholesterol diets, and improved medical services might produce new reductions in susceptibility to disease or new increases in the vigor factor.

Another method of increasing the vigor factor might be use of drugs or pharmacological agents which are not specific treatments for specific diseases, as antibiotics are, but which have more generalized effects on bodily vigor. Sacher has reviewed the experimental work with such drug treatments on mice and other small animals, and finds that they do increase the vigor factor, thus lengthening the average lifespan of these animals. However, such treatments have not yet been shown to affect the mean lifespan in man, although several substances are now being used experimentally with humans in pursuing this goal. . . .

(3) *The problem of disability and life extension.*   A question of enormous social significance is, What will happen to the amount of physical

disability in the elderly population if an extension of life is achieved? Will there be increased need for medical care, increased need for long-term care, increased years of physical or mental disability? . . .

[We know] that, by age 50, the mortality rate is substantial and doubles every eight years. From this age on, there are increasing amounts or lengthening periods of physical disability, due mainly to increased morbidity from chronic diseases. The following diseases show increased incidence, and they tend to cause more and more disability: cardiovascular disease, cancer, cerebral accidents (stroke), arthritis, rheumatism, and failing eyesight.

In addition, there are two other major causes of disability: senility and the kinds of accidents that result in broken hips and other conditions that reduce physical mobility. Senility perhaps should be regarded as a disease entity—some form of deterioration of the brain occurs, and it may progress to a point where the person can no longer care for himself.

As a result of these various diseases and disabilities, a sizable number of persons over 75 are placed in institutions where they receive such physical and medical care and such general supervision as they need. This has been an increasing number, although the number may be stabilizing at a relatively constant proportion of the over-65 population. This group includes practically all residents of nursing homes who are over 65, and a portion (but not all) of the residents of homes for the aged. It also includes a portion of the residents of State and private mental institutions.

The total number of elderly people in need of physical care and general supervision—both in and out of institutions—is estimated at between 10% to 15% of the over-65 population, or 2.6 to 3.3 million in 1975 (U.S. Congress, Senate, 1974).

The proponents of both methods of lengthening life—changing the vigor factor, and changing the rate of aging—say that they will lengthen the active and vigorous part of life. That is, they say that by appropriate methods of treatment it is possible to stretch out the *active* and *useful* life without increasing the period of physical disability. *But the evidence for this proposition is scant, whether it be related to one method or the other.* [Italics added—HJW]

It seems reasonable to suppose that with more effective methods of preventing or curing chronic diseases, older people will retain their physical activity and vigor longer. For example, if hypertension and other forms of cardiovascular disease are reduced, the physical disabilities connected with these diseases will be reduced, and people will live longer without any net increase in the amount of disability. On the other hand the disabilities attached to arthritis, rheumatism, and failing eyesight may increase as people live longer, and new treatments will be needed to reduce their incidence.

The proponents of the rate control method of extending life say that if all the living cells of the body age more slowly, the body will stay fit for a longer period. Thus a person who is 90 years old but who has undergone treatment to slow down the rate of aging will be as vigorous at 90 as he would otherwise be at age 75. His eyesight will not deteriorate as fast as it would under present-day conditions, his teeth will hold out longer, and his arthritis will not be as painful. Yet the 90-year-old will be subject to the "accidental" causes of disability, such as infections and accidents, and these will require health care and medical treatment.

Sacher argues that there is nothing in the theory of action of antiaging drugs to indicate that a reduced rate of aging will be accompanied by a reduction in morbidity, or in the average duration of time a person stays alive with a terminal disease. It seems reasonable to believe that the amount of medical care and health service needed by a particular elderly subgroup is bound to increase with the age of that subgroup, no matter what kind of antiaging treatment or preventive health care it has received. The amount of disability and dependence upon care by others is sure to be higher for the oldest 10% of the population than for younger age cohorts, and if the last survivors live more years, as they clearly do . . . they will in all probability require a greater total amount of health care and service.

It is difficult to believe that the average length of life after 65 could be extended by either of these methods without a substantial increase in the number of visits to the doctor or dentist, the number of days in the hospital, and the number of nursing home beds.

From these considerations it appears that, above all, we need more studies of the physical vigor and the health care of the population beyond age 80 or 85. Among other things, we need to examine the kinds of preventive health care and treatment persons receive after age 40 or 50.

We may be fairly sure that the average lifespan beyond age 65 will be increased by the year 2000, whether it be by two years or five years or fifteen years. Many more people will live into their 80's and 90's, and their health and happiness will be influenced by research in biogerontology. (pp. 15–18)

Editor's Bridging Comment

There are additional factors of logistical and "human nature" consideration that provide persuasive arguments against a biological resolution of the problem of aging "in our time." The first is the bottleneck in talent. There are, in any society, a limited number of people with the ability to undertake major intellectual tasks. This manpower pool may be extended with more training facilities, fellowships, and so on, but these rare individuals are required in many areas, all of which will compete for top talent, as Goddard (1977) shows.

Extension of the Lifespan: A National Goal?

J. Goddard

Changes in Biomedical Research Programs

If life extension were to be adopted as a national goal, the most immediate changes would involve our current biomedical programs with respect to research and training programs. We have in recent years substantially increased the funding for research and training related to the first three causes of death—diseases of the heart, malignant neoplasms, and cerebrovascular accidents. Our findings in these three areas account for almost 50% of our current total health research investment, but in terms of what is spent on health care services (an estimated $94 billion in 1973), it is a fairly modest amount. To have a reasonable chance of reaching the goal by the year 2000, it may be necessary to expend as much as $25 billion in total, or slightly less than the amount spent by the space agency in its program to put man on the moon.

Could we expend funds at this level and not adversely affect the efforts to discover causes of heart disease, cancer, and stroke? It seems doubtful that both efforts could be sustained at such high levels, especially during the early years—not from the point of view of impact on the national budget, but because we are limited largely by the availability of qualified persons to conduct the necessary research. Many of the persons now involved in cancer and cardiovascular research would be the very ones most needed in the new effort. It would therefore be essential in the early phases to underwrite a very substantial training program, beginning at the college level and extending through pre- and postdoctoral levels. Only through substantial investment, perhaps as much as $5 billion over the next ten to twenty years, could enough personnel become available to implement the research program at an optimal level.

To minimize the disruption in both research and training, an assessment of our resource allocation would be required which would permit a redefinition of priorities in light of the new goal; the identification of current programs and projects which fit within the new scheme of priorities; the exposition of areas requiring research effort; the definition of short- and long-range manpower requirements; the matching up of capabilities and interests of organizations and individuals with the tasks to be performed; and the institution of a management system which would couple an appropriate degree of monitoring sensitivity with the capability for periodic reassessment and redefinition of tasks. (p. 23)

Editor's Bridging Comment

In addition, we like to pretend that health and vigor are salient values for people. One look at statistics of alcoholism, obesity, tobacco smoking, dangerous driving of vehicles and such can dispel that fiction. About all that is true for most people is that we value our health most when we are ill and that we don't bother much about our health when we are well. Hayflick (1977) states the problem starkly:

[One might ask] whether any method shown to increase human longevity will, in fact, be used. The notion that any method guaranteed to reduce illness or extend life would not be used may at first seem to be naive, but we are, nonetheless, surrounded by that reality. Consider poliomyelitis and its tragic consequence. Even with the availability of a highly effective prophylaxis in what surely must be considered to be the most painless form of administration (one drop of a sweet-tasting solution on the tongue), fully 40% of preschool age children in this country are not immunized. When the vaccine first became available, long lines of people waited for treatment. The current apathy is due largely to the fact that, unlike the older generation, young adults have never seen a polio victim. Consequently, a strong motivation to voluntarily immunize their children is lacking, and were it not for the legal requirement that immunization is necessary for school admission, the likelihood is that immunization against polio would fade to zero in a few years. In order to maintain a proper level of motivation to immunize, the best method probably would be to allow a sufficient number of crippled polio victims to hobble around the streets as constant reminders of the threat. Perhaps it would be more humane to secretly employ paid actors for this purpose.

It would be my guess that like the one example cited of the many that could be given, any regimen designed to increase longevity, even one as simple as a drop of sweet-tasting fluid on the tip of the tongue, would fail one generation after its initial use. Quite obviously if no one ever saw an aged individual the likelihood is nil that he could be persuaded that for lack of treatment he might age. (p. 4)

Recommended Readings

Federation of American Societies for Experimental Biology, Session I:"Theoretical Aspects of Developmental and Age Changes." *Federation Proceedings* 34 (January 1974):5–20.

French, C. and Hayflick, L., eds. *Handbook of the Biology of Aging*. New York: Van Nostrand, 1977.

Hayflick, L. "The Strategy of Senescence." *Gerontologist* 19 (1979):37–45.

Sacher, G. "Longevity, Aging and Death: an Evolutionary Perspective." *Gerontologist*, 18 (1978):112–19.

Part Three

The Psychological Dimension

4

Aging and Intelligence

The following anecdote was contributed by Mrs. Mamie Chaif-fetz, activity therapist for the chronic brain syndrome floors at the Philadelphia Hospital and Home for the Jewish Aged. To understand the anecdote, the reader must be aware of the fact that a research project is presently under way at the home. The incident described is further documentation for the well-known fact that the interviewer and the interview influence the responses.

Mrs. R. caught me as I came out of Mrs. K.'s room and asked me to come with her into her room as she had something important to discuss with me. I followed her and she took me to the far corner of her room pulling me close to her.

Mrs. R.: You know how busy I am. How I work at two jobs for you and I do them well. And how I work for my Bertha on Tuesdays? And how busy I am in my room and clean a little and sew buttons on my clothes, and do a few repairs? And how my children visit me and I am busy with them, and sometimes I visit them? So with all I have to do, I don't have time for the president.

M. C.: That's right, so . . .

Mrs. R.: So . . . with all I have to do, and you know I am very busy. I know my name and where I am and all my children and grandchildren so how could I remember the president's name? So I forgot his name for the moment so please tell me his name again.

M. C.: His name is Johnson. Why?

Mrs. R.: That's right! Wait just a minute and I will write it down in Jewish. (This she proceeded to do as I had some qualms about having told her.)

M. C.: Why do you want to know the name of the president?

Mrs. R.: I'll tell you, because you are my friend, but don't tell anyone else. There is a sort of crazy looking man walking around and giving tests to everyone, and I worried about it. So I followed him around and listened while he asked his questions. And like I told you, I know my name and my children's names and where I am; but I didn't know the president's name and I wanted to get a good score on my test, so now I have the name written down and when he comes to me I will look at the name and give him the answer and I will get a good mark! (At this she laughed with glee and poked her elbow in my ribs, for it was obvious, she was aware that she had outsmarted the establishment.)

Mamie Chaiffetz, untitled article, *Gerontologist*

Editor's Introduction

In the past, employing largely cross-sectional studies, the evidence seemed clear that intelligence declined with advancing age. In recent years, other methods have been employed and the findings are more equivocal. An almost acrimonious debate on the subject between Paul B. Baltes and K. Warner Shaie versus John L. Horn and Gary Donaldson has taken place in the pages of *The American Psychologist* (Baltes and Schaie, 1976; Horn and Donaldson, 1976, 1977; Schaie and Baltes, 1977). Since these papers are highly technical, they are not presented in this volume. Counterarguments to the view that intelligence does not decline with age will be summarized following the presentation of Baltes' and Schaie's optimistic paper in *Psychology Today*, written in that journal's more popular style.

Whenever an "optimistic" view of no decline in function with age appears, it should be examined with more than usual care. The seductiveness of the belief in long-lived inhabitants of the several Shangri-Las has already been noted in these pages. Similar emotions about human finitude influence investigators studying the problem of decline in mental function in the aged.

> There are powerful reasons for wanting to believe that intellectual decrement does not occur. . . . Humans have a well-developed ability for wishful thinking, and most humans who derive their livelihood and status from exercise of their intellectual abilities have a strong wish that these abilities will not wane. This includes most people who do research on aging. Most of us do not desire to see our friends and loved ones lose qualities which often include their abilities. The audience for abilities research is thus set to hear what it wants to hear, and what it wants to hear is that intelligence does not decline with age. Researchers operate under a variety of subtle pressures to give this audience what it wants. This not only shapes the nature of research—the choice of variables and methods of analysis, for example—but also the interpretations given to results. (Horn and Donaldson, 1976, p. 702)

The Myth of the Twilight Years

P. B. Baltes and K. W. Schaie

News reporters never tire of pointing out that Golda Meir works 20-hour days, yet is in her mid-70s, and a grandmother. *Time*, in a recent story on William O. Douglas, noted that the blue eyes of the 75-year-old Justice "are as keen and alert as ever. So, too, is his intellect." This sort of well-intended but patronizing compliment betrays a widespread assumption that intelligence normally declines in advanced adulthood and old age, and that people like Meir and Douglas stand out as exceptions.

In our opinion, general intellectual decline in old age is largely a myth. During the past 10 years, we and our colleagues (particularly G. V. Labouvie and J. R. Nesselroade), have worked to gain a better understanding of intelligence in the aged. Our findings challenge the stereotyped view, and promote a more optimistic one. We have discovered that the old man's boast, "I'm just as good as I ever was," may be true, after all.

The Data on Decline

For a long time, the textbook view coincided with the everyday notion that as far as intelligence is concerned, what goes up must come down. The research that supported this view was cross-sectional in nature. The investigator administered intelligence tests to people of various ages at a given point in time, and compared the performance levels of the different age groups. Numerous studies of this type conducted during the '30s, '40s, and '50s led researchers to believe that intelligence increases up to early adulthood, reaches a plateau that lasts for about ten years, and begins to decline in a regular fashion around the fourth decade of life.

The first doubts arose when the results of longitudinal studies began to be available. In this type of study, the researcher observes a single group of subjects for a period of time, often extending over many years, and examines their performance at different ages. Early longitudinal studies suggested that intelligence during maturity and old age did not decline as soon as people had originally assumed.

As better intelligence tests became available, researchers began to realize that different intellectual measures might show different rates of decline. On measures of vocabulary and other skills reflecting educational experience, individuals seemed to maintain their adult level of functioning into the sixth, and even the seventh decade.

Resolving the Discrepancy

In 1956, one of us (Schaie) launched a major project aimed at resolving this disturbing discrepancy between the two kinds of study. Five hundred subjects, ranging in age from 20 to 70 received two intelligence tests, Thurstone and Thurstone's Primary Mental Abilities, and Schaie's Test of Behavioral Rigidity. Seven years later, we retested 301 of the subjects with the same tests (Schaie, 1965).

The tests we used yielded thirteen separate measures of cognitive functioning. Using factor-analysis methods, we found that the scores reflected four general, fairly independent dimensions of intelligence: (1) Crystallized intelligence encompasses the sorts of skills one acquires through education and acculturation, such as verbal comprehension, numerical skills, and inductive reasoning. To a large degree, it reflects the extent to which one has accumulated the collective intelligence of one's own culture. It is the dimension tapped by most traditional IQ tests (Cattell, March, 1958). (2) Cognitive flexibility measures the ability to shift from one way of thinking to another, within the context of familiar intellectual operations, as when one must provide either an antonym or synonym to a word, depending on whether the word appears in capital or lower-case letters. (3) Visuo-motor flexibility measures a similar, but independent skill, the one involved in shifting from familiar to unfamiliar patterns in tasks requiring coordination between visual and motor abilities, e.g., when one must copy words but interchange capitals with lower-case letters. (4) Finally visualization measures the ability to organize and process visual materials and involves tasks such as finding a simple figure contained in a complex one or identifying a picture that is incomplete. The Schaie study did not contain sufficient measures of fluid intelligence, which encompasses abilities thought to be relatively culture free. Other researchers, e.g., Cattell and Horn (Horn and Cattell, 1966, 1967), have reported a dramatic decline with age on fluid intelligence, though on the basis of cross-sectional data only.

If we analyze the data cross-sectionally (comparing the different age groups at a given point in time), we get the conventional pattern of early, systematic decline. But when we look at the results longitudinally (comparing a given age group's performance in 1956 with its performance in 1963), we find a definite decline on only one of the four measures, visuomotor flexibility (Baltes, 1968).

There is no strong age-related change in cognitive flexibility. For the most important dimension, crystallized intelligence, and for visualization as well, we see a systematic increase in scores for the various age groups, right into old age. Even people over 70 improved from the first testing to the second.

Intellectual Generation Gap

In cross-sectional studies, people who differ in age also differ in generation, since they were born in different years. This means that any measured differences in intelligence could reflect either age or generation differences, or both. Our study, however, allowed us to compare people from different generations at the same ages, because we tested people at two different points in time. For instance, we could compare subjects who were 50 in 1956 with subjects who were 50 in 1963. Our statistical analysis revealed that the differences between scores were due mainly to generational differences, not to chronological age. In other words, the important factor was the year a subject was born, rather than his age at the time of testing. Apparently, the measured intelligence of the population is increasing. The earlier findings of general intellectual decline over the individual life span were largely an artifact of methodology. On at least some dimensions of intelligence, particularly the crystallized type, people of average health can expect to maintain or even increase their level of performance into old age (Baltes, 1968).

At present, we can only speculate about the reasons for generational differences in intelligence. We believe the answer lies in the substance, method, and length of education received by different generations. When we consider the history of our educational institutions, and census data on the educational levels attained by members of specific generations, it seems fair to assume that the older people in our study were exposed to shorter periods of formal education. Furthermore, their education probably relied more heavily on principles of memorization, and less heavily on those of problem-solving.

However, there are other possibilities that must be reckoned with before we can offer a more definite interpretation. Members of different generations may differ in their sophistication in test-taking or their willingness to volunteer responses. They may differ in the extent to which they have been encouraged to achieve intellectually. And tests developed to measure the abilities of one generation may be invalid for another. In any case, the existence of differences between generations makes the search for "normal" aging phenomena a Sisyphean task.

Drop Before Death

Klaus and Ruth Riegel (Riegel and Riegel, 1967, 1972), psychologists at the University of Michigan, have recently suggested when intellectual decline does occur, it comes shortly before death. In 1956, the Riegels gave intelligence tests to 380 German men and women between the ages of 55 and 75. Five years later they retested 202 of them. Some of the remainder had died, and others refused to be retested. When the Riegels looked back at the 1956 test scores of the subjects who had died, they discovered that on the average, the deceased subjects had scored lower than those who survived. Put another way, the low scores in 1956 predicted impending death.

The Riegels followed up their study in 1966 by inquiring into the fate of the people retested in 1961 (Riegel and Riegel, 1967). Again, some people had died in the interim, and those who had died had lower scores than those who lived. Furthermore, people who had died since 1961 had declined in score from the first test session in 1956 to the second in 1961. These results pointed to a sudden deterioration during the five or fewer years immediately prior to natural death, or what the Riegels called a "terminal drop." Interestingly, the people who had refused to be retested in 1961 were more likely than the others to die before 1966. Perhaps their refusal reflected some kind of awareness of their own decline.

The Riegels' results may offer an alternative explanation for the general decline found by cross-sectional studies: the older groups may contain a higher percentage of people in the terminal drop stage, and their lower scores would not be typical of other older people. If the researcher could foresee the future and remove from his study those subjects nearing death, he might observe little or no change in the intelligence of the remaining group. In fact, the Riegels found that elderly subjects still alive in 1966 did as well, on the average, as persons at the presumed period of peak performance, 30 to 34 years, which of course, is consistent with our own data.

While it is tempting to speculate on the reasons for terminal drop, we feel that the present state of the art is such that interpretation must be tentative at best. Most researchers would probably tend to relate the drop in intellectual functioning to neurophysiological deterioration. However, this position overlooks the possibility that psychological variables contribute both to the drop and to biological death.

Aged-Biased IQ Tests

The nature of the tests used to assess intelligence may also contribute to the apparent decline that is sometimes observed. Sidney L. Pressey (who now lives as an octogenarian in a home for the elderly and continues to make occasional but insightful contributions to psychology) first pointed out that the concept of intelligence, as well as the instruments to measure it, are defined in terms of abilities most important during youth and early adulthood (Demming and Pressey, 1957). This is not really surprising, since IQ tests came into existence for the purpose of predicting school performance. The format and content of these tests may simply be inappropriate for tapping the potential wisdom of the aged. For example, older people tend to do relatively poorly on tests employing technical language such as the terminology of physics or computer programming. Their performance is better if items are worded in terms of everyday experiences.

Another problem is the distinction between a person's competence and his actual performance. Handicaps that have nothing to do with intrinsic ability may affect the way a person does on a test. For instance, Baltes and Carol A. Furry recently demonstrated that the aged are especially susceptible to the effects of fatigue; pretest fatigue considerably lowered the scores of older subjects, but did not affect the performance of younger ones (Furry and Baltes, 1973).

Dwindling reinforcements may also affect the performance of the aged. Elderly individuals, because of their uncertain and shortened life expectancy, may cease to be sensitive to the sorts of long-range rewards that seem to control intellectual behavior in young people (e.g., education, career goals, and development of a reputation). Ogden Lindsley has proposed that the aged may become more dependent on immediate and idiosyncratic rewards.

Even when rewards are potentially effective, they may be unavailable to old people. Most researchers agree that the environment of the elderly is intellectually and socially impoverished. Family settings and institutions for the aged fail to provide conditions conducive to intellectual growth. The educational system discourages participation by the elderly, focusing instead on the young.

Recent work on age stereotypes indicates that some young people hold a negative view of old age. These views may influence them to withdraw reinforcements for competence in the elderly, or even to punish such competence. Aging persons may in time come to accept the stereotypes, view themselves as deficient, and put aside intellectual performance as a personal goal. In the process the intellectual deficit becomes a self-fulfilling prophecy.

Compensatory Education for the Aged

Although educators have made massive attempts to overcome discrimination in early childhood, working through government-funded compensatory programs, analogous efforts for the aged have barely begun. But increasing numbers of gerontologists have felt encouraged enough by the reanalysis of intellectual decline to examine, probably for the first time in any vigorous manner, the degree to which intellectual performance can be bolstered. The results are still very sketchy, but they are promising.

Some researchers, working from a bio-behavioral perspective, have looked at the effects of physical treatments. For instance, hyperbaric oxygen treatment for extended periods to increase oxygen supply to the brain, seems to improve memory for recent events, although the outcome of such research is not at all free of controversy. Treatment of hypertension and conditioning of alpha waves also seem to be promising, and deserve careful study. Other researchers concentrate on studying the psychological aspects of the learning process; they experiment with the pacing of items, the mode of presentation (for instance, auditory versus visual), the amount of practice, the delivery of rewards, training in mnemonics, and so on.

The speed with which a person responds, which is important on many intellectual tests, is usually assumed to be a function of biological well-being. But in a series of pilot studies, Baltes, William Hoyer, and Gisela V. Labouvie were able to improve the response speed of elderly subjects rather dramatically, using Green Stamps as a reward for faster performance in cancelling letters, marking answer sheets, and copying words. After as little as two hours of training, women 65 to 80 years of age increased their speed as much as 20 to 35%. The researchers compared the performance of these "trained" subjects with that of untrained controls on eleven different intellegence tests. Although the transfer of the speed training to test performance was not earthshaking, the overall pattern was encouraging (Hoyer, et al., 1973).

In the interest of rectifying some of the social injustices that have resulted from the branding of the aged as deficient, social scientists must continue to explore, with vigor and optimism, the research avenues opened during the past few years. This research should be guided by a belief in the potential of gerontological intelligence, and a rejection of the rigid, biological view that assumes an inevitable decline. We should not be surprised to find that the socialization goals and mechanisms of a society are the most powerful influence on what happens to people, not only during childhood and adolescence but also during adulthood and old age.

Social roles and resources can be assigned without regard to age only when the deleterious aspects of aging are eliminated. Toward this end, at a meeting in 1971 an American Psychological Association task force on aging made some specific recommendations for eliminating the unnecessary causes of decline in intellectual functioning (Eisdorfer and Lawton, 1973). They included more forceful implementation of adult-education programs; funding of research and innovative programs in voluntary (rather than mandatory) retirement, second-career training, and leisure-time activity; and better utilization of skills that are unaffected by age.

When we consider the vast spectrum of negative conditions, attributes, and expectations that most Western societies impose on older people, we must acclaim the impressive robustness of our older population in the face of adversity. At the same time, we hope that society, aided by gero-psychology, soon finds ways to make life for the elderly more enjoyable and effective. Acknowledging that intellectual decline is largely a myth is, we hope, a step in the right direction.

Editor's Comment

Sampling design problems. The first problem that arises in a critique of the "Myth of the Twilight Years" is that cross-sectional and longitudinal studies utilize samples from different populations and therefore arrive at different conclusions. As Baltes and Schaie suggest, older-age cohorts, on the whole, test lower. However, these generational differences account for only about 20% of test score variance. Individual differences within age groups are much greater. We will soon return to the problem of individual changes.

Longitudinal samples (testing the same sample over and over) create different problems, the least of which is probably the effect of multiple administration of similar tests. It does not seem reasonable to expect that tests given at intervals of from once a year to once in seven years create "test wiseness," that is, greater ease, sophistication, and familiarity with the material. Indeed, what happens is quite different. Those who score low initially tend both to die sooner and to refuse to participate in later retests, which latter effect Baltes and Schaie realize, but seem to ignore. The more able ones, invariably, show up for retest in greater proportions. I know of no studies that control for social class factors in dropping out; it is, however, again reasonable to expect that good test takers are more likely to be better educated, therefore to have higher incomes, access to better medical care, nutrition, housing, sanitation, and so on, and to survive for retesting. Low scorers, in addition to being of lower social class and income, with their concomitant disadvantages, are also likely to be discouraged, threatened, and humiliated by their poor performance, of which they are likely to be aware and also tend not to survive to retest. So longitudinal samples, no matter how randomly selected at first, develop with time into highly biased samples, most unrepresentative of the original sample.

The effects of bias, accumulating as successive samples are tested, is evident, as this discussion shows. Baltes and Schaie state, in their *Psychology Today* paper (1974), that

> for the most important dimension, crystalized intelligence, and for visualization as well, we see a systematic *increase* [italics in the original] in scores for various age groups, right into old age. Even people over 70 improved from the first testing to the second. (p. 36)

However, the data, when carefully analyzed, do not bear out this conclusion. Selective attrition of subjects accounts for the claimed stability and improvement of test scores. "The *means* of the 1956 scores, *but of the remaining subjects only* (N = 302) were higher than those of the total group tested in 1956 (N = 500)" (Botwinick, 1977, pp. 590–591; italics in the original), that is, those *retested* in 1963 were originally high scorers of the sample. Indeed, when a third wave of testing was done in 1970, there was a further increase in the 1956 IQ of those subjects who returned for testing the third time (N = 161).

It is also quite artificial to attempt to segregate effects of chronological aging from cohort-generational effects. It is as meaningless as attempting to separate the effects of heredity and environment. An individual with a given capacity for development matures in a certain environment; you can't "do the experiment over" of having a sample be conceived again in 1960 instead of 1900 and see how different its development will be. And it is, I hope, inconceivable that some mad scientist will someday clone a number of aged individuals in order to regrow and retest them a generation or two later. Schaie (1965) and Baltes (1968) have developed a method called sequential analysis, which attempts to add new and previously untested cohort samples at each retest of the same age as the older sample.

Even sequential analysis cannot provide a completely satisfactory solution to the problems inherent in longitudinal and cross-sectional studies. The very nature of the problem of people living in a constantly changing society introduces irreducible ambiguity in determining the effect of age and cohort in such studies. No statistical manipulation can wholly remove the cross-sectional effect of improvement in literacy, test-taking confidence, and better living conditions over the generations, and the biasing effect of selective return for retesting of the high scorers of any generation, but especially of older people (Horn and Donaldson, 1976; Botwinick, 1977).

Problems in testing older people. What Baltes and Schaie (1974) refer to as "verbal ability," "crystallized intelligence," does tend to bear up with age better than do such measures of capacity as "performance tests," cognitive or visual-motor flexibility or visualization. Items included under verbal or crystallized intelligence, such as vocabulary items, synonyms and antonyms, and inductive reasoning without associated "fancy tricks," are more frequently performed by educated, literate, white-collar people in the course of their daily lives, if not in their work then in play, for example, doing crossword puzzles. Performance, visual-motor flexibility, and visualization include more activities that are artificial to most adults who, in their daily lives, do not willingly "jump through hoops" at the behest of usually young adult psychometricians who want them to assemble Rube Goldberg objects, trace mazes, put blocks together to form patterns, and to solve mathematical problems the appropriate formulae for which they have long forgotten. In addition, older people may often feel less compulsion to please the tester and to show him or her how nimble their minds are. One of the nicer things about being old is that you have achieved whatever you are going to achieve in this world and you don't have to strive at meaningless tasks to prove anything to a young whippersnapper (Wershow, 1964). Such behavior is labelled "poor motivation."
Problems of testing of older people are further confounded by factors such as: old people tend to tire more easily than younger; they may need breaks or have the test administered in two sessions; they also tend to do poorly in time-limited tests. However, *younger people improve even more than the old* when time limits are ignored and older people, while they benefit by ignoring time limits, do not reach the high performance levels of younger people in performance

tests. Some of the differences between younger and older subjects'
test scores are attributable to health.

> Health related differences are no more mythical when they are
> associated with persons of different ages than when they are associ-
> ated with persons of the same age but of different social classes or
> different disease histories. It does not aid the understanding or the
> treatment of such conditions (if they exist) to refer to associated
> differences as mythical. Indeed, even if all age differences were
> shown unequivocally to indicate generational differences, and this
> alone, the differences would be no less real, and there would be no
> less need to seek understanding of these differences in terms of
> factors of health and hygiene and experience. Also, it must be noted
> that when special efforts are made to sample only particularly healthy
> older persons, the universe of generalization of results based on such
> sampling is not that of adults, qua adults, as is implied in arguments
> that decrement is a myth. (Horn and Donaldson, 1976, p. 707)

The aged are certainly more likely to experience ill health,
impending death, and possible "terminal drop" which add to the
chances of greater intellectual deficit with aging. But all these
factors are part of aging in the real world, not alone in the laboratory.
Other studies show that both performance and verbal scores decline
in later life, after age 60–70. Those with higher mental abilities also
decline, though the decline from an IQ of 160 to 130 may be less
noticeable than a decline from 100 to 70. Botwinick (1977) summa-
rizes the findings on decline in intelligence thusly:

> A summary of the cross-sectional literature suggests that the age-
> intelligence relationship tends to be small, with decline not setting in
> until relatively late in life. [that is, decline begins in the 50s or
> 60s—HJW] Longitudinal studies, while accurately reflecting
> changes among those people available for retesting, do not accurately
> reflect changes of more complete populations. . . . When the limita-
> tions of the cohort effect in cross-sectional research and the selective
> dropout effect in longitudinal research are recognized, the two
> methods may provide similar interpretations; differences are quan-
> titative, not qualitative. (pp. 589, 591, and 603)

Age-related differences are greater and occur earlier than the
50s or 60s in tasks involving speed of response of nonverbal, percep-

tual manipulative skills. Beyond these observations, the detailed results are complex. Those interested in further details are referred to papers in the bibliography at the end of this chapter.

The effect of training on test scores. Whether training improves test scores is largely irrelevant to the argument. Training may very well increase scores of younger subjects who lack opportunities for the skills and knowledge that training improves.

This is not to argue that intervention research of the kind outlined above is not valuable or does not help to deal with intellectual deficits. Indeed, when a condition of deficit is shown to exist, it is precisely such research which can provide the means for effective amelioration. One of the major points of this paper is that the basis for launching such desirable research is not improved by referring to evidence for deficit as myth. (Horn and Donaldson, 1976, p. 705)

Editor's Conclusion

In general, the polemic cited is useful in that it reminds us that *"the aged"* is as pernicious a concept as are *"the* black man," *"the* oppressed female half of the world" and other counter-stereotypic stereotypes. Among older people, women, blacks, and other minority and quasiminority groups there exist large within-group differences, on any and all attributes, usually larger than mean differences between groups. For the rest, Schaie and Baltes protest in their replies (Baltes and Schaie, 1976; Schaie and Baltes, 1977) that they never claimed there were *no* differences of consequence, merely that the differences are not invariant, that they are multidimensional and multidirectional, and that a stance of denying deficits will lead to a more hopeful attitude, more vigorous research, and focus on the plasticity of adult and gerontological behavior.

We would suggest that future research be directed to these questions:

1. So what? What effect does decline in one element of intellectual functioning or another have upon coping ability? How much of which of these factors is most necessary to get along in a complex

urban environment, and are these the factors that decline more rapidly in more people?

2. If we can pinpoint the disabilities that hamper functioning in society, can they be compensated? Can certain environmental aspects be modified to enable those with certain functional deficits to remain independent and relatively content with their lives? Can intervention techniques be developed that compensate for or reverse lost function?

Few studies attempt to make the transition from the test situation to real situations, from the laboratory to life. Without providing much evidence for his beliefs, Schaie (1974) asserts that adult education programs, possibly with compulsory features (with truant officers and "please excuse my father from school today" letters?), variable retirement policies, and diminishing age-segregated living will help our older citizens. These may be desirable steps to undertake, but the "scientific base" for such policy decisions is far from well-established.

Recommended Readings

Botwinick, J. "Intelligence." In *Aging and Behavior,* 2d rev. ed., edited by J. Botwinick. New York: Springer, 1978, pp. 208–33.

Jarvick, L.; Eisdorfer, C.; and Blum, J., eds. *Intellectual Functioning in Adults.* New York: Springer, 1973. See especially the chapter by C. Eisdorfer and F. Wilkie, "Intellectual Changes with Advancing Age," pp. 21–79.

5

The Theory of Disengagement

I could be well content
To entertain the lag end of my life
With quiet hours.

Shakespeare, *King Henry IV, Part I*

Editor's Introduction

It is unfortunate that, to our knowledge, no one or two relatively short and nontechnical papers have appeared that can be used to summarize the ongoing disputation around the theory of disengagement. This presentation is largely drawn from several papers, noted in the appended Bibliography. The major value of disengagement theory is that it forced the field of gerontology to look beyond the simplistic, often implicit, previously unquestioned and taken for granted "activity" theory, which assumed that "successful" aging (however defined and measured) necessitated maintaining life styles and activity that duplicate, as much as possible, those of adults of preretirement age and status.

Disengagement theory is of importance because it is the first attempt to describe the aging process in terms other than pious exhortations to "wear out, not rust out," deprecations of the "rocking chair on the front porch" syndrome, though even that can be a form of engagement, as is evidenced by Lozier and Althouse (1975). Disengagement theory recognizes that frenetic activity may not necessarily be the healthiest way to age; it takes into account the reality that many older people may not have the reserves of physical, emotional, even intellectual energy to be as involved, committed, zestfully engaged in hobbies, family life, community activity (if not employment) as are people in mid-career. In short, disengagement theory entertains the possibility that older people may be different than younger people in some ways.

Definition of disengagement. The idea that society and the aging individual engage in a mutual process of disengagement arose from an almost serendipitious finding in the Kansas City studies (Cumming and Henry, 1961). This research involved 257 people, ranging in age from 50 to 90, all of whom were in good health and financially independent. While such a population omits the sick, poor elderly, it is useful precisely because it makes it possible to study the effects of aging uncontaminated by the additional influence of poverty and illness (Wershow, 1969, 1973a).

Unexpectedly, as subjects aged and many withdrew from activity, their scores on measurements of "morale," "well-being," and "life-satisfaction" did not necessarily decline. Indeed, the theory claims to be neutral as to the relationship between disengagement and happiness of the aged. Rather, the theory explains disengagement process as intrinsic to and necessary for aging as is the loss of the thymus gland as children develop. Happiness is as unrelated to disengagement as it is to loss of that tissue.

The theory contains several propositions:

1.   The life space of an individual decreases with age, in that he or she interacts with a narrower variety of role partners and spends a smaller proportion of his or her time in interaction. This proposition was later elaborated to highlight the importance of vacating the key life roles of work and family.

2.   The individual anticipates this change and participates in the process.

3.   The individual's preference for interpersonal rewards becomes more individualized and expressive, and less role-connected as he or she grows older, and thus the style of interaction changes.

4.   Once begun, the process is irreversible. As the individual relinquishes obligatory roles, he or she is unlikely to either seek out or be sought out for new obligatory roles, because the person gains freedom as he or she loses centrality in the social order and society gains the possibility of circulation of statuses; the young have the opportunity to move up.

5.   When the process of disengagement is completed, the individual has given up the equilibrium that characterized middle

age and achieves a new equilibrium based on greater social and psychological distance and fewer and more superficial relationships between self and society.

Disengagement takes place in both the social and normative realms, i.e., both in interaction with others and in the values one assigns to those interactions. In the social realm:

1. Roles are reduced to exclude those that endow the person with power and important social roles. Remaining roles are often limited to emotional-affective components, for example, the role of grandparent instead of parent of a not-yet independent child.

2. The social network of the individual tends to decrease to a small social circle of immediate family, kin, neighbors, and old friends. Relationships in the work place and larger associations are lost or diminished.

3. Older people tend to live in a segregated subculture of the aged.

4. Relationships tend to be more shallow and superficial than were earlier relationships.

In the normative realm:

1. As the changes in the social realm progress, the individual is progressively freed from the constraints of informal social controls.

2. Idiosyncratic behavior increases as social controls diminish.

3. As the society is relatively unaffected by behavior of the disengaged, it tends to be indifferent to these idiosyncratic behaviors.

4. As activity of the disengaged tend to be unrelated to accomplishment and the attendant social approbation, enjoyment in activity is diminished (adapted from Cumming, 1963, 1975).

Normative and social engagement may vary independently with age. They may be positively or inversely related to each other, for a person can ritualistically maintain a broad spectrum of associations that have long been robbed of inner importance or meaning. According to Hochschild (1975) there is also psychological disengagement that is,

> as later research suggests, probably related to nearness of death and may not be of crucial importance until the last years. Before the very final years, I would suggest that psychological engagement is a consequence of normative disengagement. Research has shown that psychological disengagement can precede social disengagement. It has not been shown to precede normative disengagement (e.g., a loss of meaning in work). . . . (p. 563)
>
> Furthermore, Cumming and Henry assumed that nearness to death and awareness of death were crucial for some twenty-five or thirty years prior to death. But Lieberman and Coplan (1970) found that those in their study who were two years away from death did show the telltale signs of disengagement, while those who were not two years away from death, did not. Their study suggests that disengagement may be closer to a two-year than a twenty-five or thirty-year process. (p. 559)

It is no exaggeration to state that the theory implies that both society and the aged person prepare for his or her death by this process of mutual withdrawal, of loosening of ties in emotional investment, life space, and time in worldly affairs. This is the function of disengagement; neither society nor the person are overly disturbed by the person's leaving, which then hurts neither party too much. Indeed, Cumming (1963) tells us the amount of disruption that would follow a person's sudden death is a measure of the depth and breadth of his or her disengagement.

The theory of disengagement may be summarized as follows:

> In every culture and historical period, the society and the individual prepare in advance for the ultimate disengagement of death by an inevitable, gradual and mutually satisfying process of social disengagement prior to death. This is a double withdrawal from society and society from the individual. . . . The remaining relationships are, in addition, qualitatively different (i.e. more socio-emotional and expressive). . . . Once set in motion, the process is irreversible. . . . This process is functional for the individual in the sense that it goes

with having a high morale, and it is functional for society in that it
retires an age echelon from roles which young people may fill. . . .
The process is universal and inevitable. (Hochschild, 1975, p. 553)

Critical analysis of disengagement theory. Disengagement
theory is an attempt to refute the common assumptions of "geroac-
tivism." It raises some very pertinent issues. For example, why
should an aged person with high "morale" necessarily need to be
useful to those around him or her? Why should it not be perfectly
acceptable to be relieved that one no longer must be useful? "It has
seldom been suggested," Cumming and Henry (1961) note, "that
people past 60 are glad to quit some of their activities. . . . Why is it
not suggested instead that old people may want recognition for
having *been* useful, for a *history* of successful instrumentality?" (p.
20). These authors wonder why aging is seen as a constant struggle
(with the approbation of the world) to maintain a middle-aged state
of equilibrium, rather than to *shift* to the equilibrium appropriate to
that stage of the life cycle. The shift from childhood to adolescence is
more poignant than the loss of middle age, but is rarely so noted,
except for some few perceptive writers of fiction. Is it perhaps a
dawning of recognition of the privileges of older people, who can
exercise their eccentricities and individualities without reproach,
that aging is perhaps not wholly euphemistically called the "golden
age"?

Cumming and Henry (1961) see disengagement flowing out of
the anticipation of death, therefore leading to "a mutual severing of
ties between a person and others in his society" (p. 211). Because
disengagement leads to a decrease in roles and a lessening of the
quality of relationships, the disengaging person is less bound by the
norms of everyday behavior. This growing idiosyncracy and eccen-
tricity leads to increasing rejection by others and a self-perpetuating
cycle of withdrawal. Disengagement is functional to our society
because "the young must be trained and the old retired before their
knowledge is obsolete" (p. 213) by the impersonal and nonjudgmen-
tal mechanism of age-grading, that is, one's time has come to retire
from work, from leadership in voluntary associations, from active
control over one's children. People who perceive their life span's
finitude, their life space decreasing and ego-energy lessened, are
ready to disengage, which coincides with society's needs. For the

powerful of society, this process may be more traumatic than it is to other people.

?78

Critical analysis of uses of the theory. It is most probably true that propositions 1 and 3 above (p. 64) do occur. Older people do, as a rule, lose roles, many are "more individualized and expressive" in their "preference for interpersonal roles," and the "style of interaction" of many aged does change. The controversy is about the inevitability and mutuality of the process and the individual's "anticipation" of and "participation" in it. The issue has also been beclouded by side issues, of the relationship between "happiness," illness, and disengagement. The major difference between disengagement and inactivity is that disengagement necessarily involves neither activity nor inactivity, isolation nor a greater number of relationships. Disengagement entails emotional uninvolvement and a withdrawal of commitment to roles and activities. Unfortunately, the Kansas City studies collected no data on feelings, but inferred them from activity and number of roles in which subjects partook (Hochschild, 1975). The original data for the theory were, then, inadequate to test its validity. Maddox (1969) presents evidence from another longitudinal study conducted at Duke University that confirms that disengagement does occur, but questions its intrinsic nature and inevitability. Streib (1964) presents evidence that to him is abundant evidence of the universality of disengagement, which he claims is a biological and social-psychological process present in all societies. His interpretation of phenomena as disengagement, however, seems to us deficient and subject to other interpretations. Streib quotes Simmons (1945) who tells us that, in preliterate societies, old people are more active in complex ceremonies and rituals that make use of their lifelong experience, as well as doing more of the lighter tasks of the group than they performed in the time of greater physical vigor.

Since teaching and performing ceremonials and rituals are considered vital functions and the performers are highly revered in these societies, can one legitimately claim lack of emotional involvement and commitment of these walking encyclopedias, prayer books, and manuals of discipline? Simmons then discusses abandonment of the elderly in some "primitive" groups as an ultimate form of disengagement. Abandonment of the aged to die on the way to the next camp is a matter of dire necessity. If the group is slowed down and cannot arrive at the next water hole in time, the entire unit will die. What has this to do with narrowing variety of role partners, decreased life space, the individual's anticipation of and participation in the process of disengagement? It is a matter of survival of the group, and of little applicability and comparability to any modern society. Streib then gives examples from rural France and Ireland, which evidence no more than, as small landholders become physically unable to work on the farm (which is the crucial variable, related to but somewhat independent of age), they give up the management role to a son, if the latter has remained at home long enough to take on the job. These are examples of loss of physical function in a society that demands hard physical labor. The previously noted "wise man of the group" in nomadic groups can carry on no longer. He must be sacrificed, not disengaged, when he can no longer ambulate. In another example of disengagement in a French village, a peasant replied matter of factly, in answer to a farewell statement of an anthropologist that they would meet again when he returned on his next sabbatical, that he was already 71 years old and not too many people of that age can look ahead to meetings that far in the future. Is meeting reality head-on and courageously "disengagement"? So much of what passes as evidence for disengagement is, at best, questionable corroboration of the theory. The experimental evidence, like much social science experimentation, adds little to our knowledge about disengagement. Experiments operationalize their definitions idiosyncratically, use different measuring instruments, and are, in short, rarely cumulative.

Basic defects in the theory.   But as Hochschild (1975) points out, there are basic defects in the theory itself. The criteria for explicating disengagement are such that nothing older people do can be used as evidence against it; people who do not conform to the theory are merely characterized as "unsuccessful" disengagers. The possibility that they may successfully remain engaged is not considered as an alternative. Cases that do not fit the theory can be dismissed as "off on their timing," but still on the way to disengagement, or they can be anomalous elitists, that is, freaks who refuse to develop properly. Or if they have passionate interests—Henry

(1964) belittles an enthusiastic chinchilla breeder as "unassertive emotionally and voyeuristic" (p. 26)—they can be variously explained away. As Hochschild (1975) states, "we do not need more replications of an unfalsifiable theory but a theory with clear criteria for counter evidence" (p. 557). Another problem is that both independent variables, age and society's permission to disengage, and the dependent variable, disengagement, have many complex intervening variables that modify their interrelationships and that crowd together, under one umbrella, many distinct phenomena—personality, sex role, life situation (which itself encompasses such categories as class, race, religion). The various dimensions of disengagement spawn "dozens of distinct dependent variables" of which "former parts of these whole variables can be transformed into promising new independent variables" and so on (Hochschild, 1975, p. 557).

It can be successfully argued that

> There are existential necessities that impinge on most men, especially in later life—the exigencies of illness, of failing strength, of approaching death, of reduced opportunity and hope—that are independent of specific cultural circumstances just as they may be independent of any prior psychological or developmental events. These existential imperatives may be the independent variables, the independent engines of psychological change in later life. (Hochschild, 1975, p. 559)

Just as long term unemployment leads to

> social and psychological disengagement among young unemployed men . . . the same can be said for old men who are forced to retire. Thus, it is not age per se, but involuntary economic disengagement itself which fosters passive and magical mastery, a loss of affect intensity—the hallmarks of "successful" psychological disengagement. (Hochschild, 1975, pp. 559–560).

If role loss can be separated from what remains of the indicators of disengagement, age as an independent variable disappears.

When
role loss (that is, widowhood, poor health, and retirement) is held
constant, the relationship between age and disengagement disappears. In their partial correlations between engagement measures,
age and role loss, they found that even with age partialled out, the
association between disengagement and role loss remained. In fact,
when the association between age and role loss was partialled out, the
link between age and disengagement dropped to zero. (Hochschild,
1975, p. 559)

The irrefutability of disengagement theory is indicated by
Hochschild in two examples well worth quoting.

In *Growing Old* (Cumming and Henry, 1961), a woman described as
"active" is said to be in a role "appropriate to the disengaged state" (p.
158). This may be a good characterization of her role—horizontal,
somewhat fragile, and temporary. But how do we characterize an
active person in a disengaged role? Consider the following case: a
woman finds that her lifelong friends and her spouse have died. She
moves into a public housing project for older people, goes to meetings, finds new friends, and takes up some new hobbies with these
new friends, one of whom she is seriously thinking of marrying.
Cumming and Henry would point out that her new relationships do
not compare in depth to her former ones, that this stage of reengage-
ment is to be temporary. But what evidence is there, apart from the
fact that her friends are necessarily new, that the woman is not asking
of her new relationships what she asked of her former ones? In such a
case, the decision of whether to characterize her as merely "active" or
as "engaged" rests on what she wants from these relationships that
she also wanted from earlier ones. Disengagement is defined by the
character of an actor's relationships to people. One dimension of a
relationship is the actor's own conscious feelings about it. If the actor
consciously feels committed or wants to feel committed to another
person and is also socially active in her behavior, I think we can
characterize her as "engaged." If she happens to die the next day, she
can be said to have died in the engaged state. . . .
     Presuming for the moment that social interaction does decrease
with age, how do we know that normative control automatically
decreases as well? Is it reasonable to assume that a 60-year-old adult,
capable of experiencing guilt for violations invisible to others, is

normatively controlled in proportion to the number of visitors he or she has each week? Is it reasonable to assume that all eccentric behavior is due to a lack of normative control? The causal links here depend on the actor's construction of reality. In my own study (Hochschild, 1973), eccentric behavior (wearing diamond earrings and tight slacks in the recreation room) was due more to a resistance to acknowledged normative control than due to the absence of it. This resident told me that she "liked getting a rise" out of her more conventional midwestern neighbors. She knew and cared what they thought. She was not de-socialized; she was just eccentric. I know this because I asked her directly. (Hochschild, 1975, p. 561)

Revisions of the theory. Hochschild suggests that disengagement may be characteristic of an industrial society. In subsistence agricultural or nomadic preindustrial societies, land and other wealth was owned or controlled by the elders; in a nonmarket economy with few labor-saving devices, neither adolescence nor aging are "social problems" (indeed, there were few who lived beyond age 40–50); all hands were needed and all were useful. In postindustrial society, large proportions of both old and young may choose not to work (or be herded onto reservations called "higher education" or "senior centers," which, while not honorific, are no great disgrace either). Industrial society, with its base in assembly line heavy industry, uses brawny youth but rejects the aged, while making a virtue of the work ethic as the basis for worth. Middle-class professionals, in both industrial and postindustrial society, may disengage less and/or later. Working class males may retain their masculine roles as being intermediary between the home and outside world and/or by broadening their engagement as father-husband. These are options alternative to disengagement. Hochschild has admittedly not attempted to deal with older women's engagement problems nor the relationship between social-normative and psychological disengagement. She does, however, make a forceful case for breaking down the global hypothesis of disengagement into subhypotheses that are applicable to both sexes, people living in different socioeconomic worlds and life styles, "until we find some [hypotheses] that work empirically in the social and phenomenological worlds of old people" (Hochschild, 1975, p. 567).

Cumming (1975) attempts to break down the all-embracing

nature and therefore unassailability of disengagement theory by differentiating between styles of disengagement that differ by temperament. She postulates "impinging" and "selecting" modes of disengagement. Every person has a more or less stable self-concept or self-image, which he or she tries to maintain intact. Impingers select out their interaction with other responses that confirm their self-concept. If responses are inappropriate to this goal, they try to change others' views of them to meet their self-image. Only if they fail repeatedly will they reluctantly modify their self-concept, and presumably their behavior. Impingers may be roughly classifiable with Reisman's "inner-directed" people (1950). Selectors, by contrast, are less aggressive or manipulative in their relations with others. They hold back and wait for others to respond in ways they deem appropriate. They select cues that meet their expectations and equally reluctantly (for it is a property of this misanthropic species to hold on to its sense of dignity and self-worth) attempt to change their concepts to bring them into line with external reality (unlike the impinger, who tries to change the others' perception), that is, to be "other-directed."

Selectors are likely to be seen by others as "reserved," "self-sufficient," or "stubborn," while impingers receive more outgoing characterizations by others as "temperamental," "brash," or "lively." Of course, Cumming (1963) recognizes that temperament is multidimensional and normally distributed, with few people at either extreme.

> The disengaging impinger can be expected to be more active and apparently more youthful than his peers. His judgment may not be as good as it was, but he will provoke the comment that he is an unusual person for his age. Ultimately, as he becomes less able to control the situation he provokes, he may suffer anxiety and panic through failure both to arouse and to interpret appropriate reactions. His problem in old age will be to avoid confusion.
>
> The selector, in contrast to the impinger, interacts in a more measured way. When he is young he may be thought too withdrawn, but as he grows older his style becomes more age-appropriate. In old age, because of his reluctance to generate interaction, he may, like a neglected infant, develop a kind of marasmus. His foe will be apathy rather than confusion.
>
> These are not, of course, ordinary aging processes; the extreme

impinger and the extreme selector are almost certain to get into trouble at some crisis point because they cannot move over to the opposite mode of interacting when it is adaptive to do so. (Cumming, 1963, pp. 380–381)

If social scientists paid more attention to the principle of Ockham's Razor (Russell, 1945), there might be fewer grand theories spun out of gossamer and we might have a greater tendency to stick to reality. Ockham's Razor postulates that, given the choice of theories, the one with the fewest basic assumptions is more likely to be true. As Hochschild has pointed out earlier, disengagement is the dependent variable, related not so much to age and society's attitude toward the aged, as it is to role losses such as widowhood and retirement and to ill health. It is inevitable, because there are "the existential necessities that impinge . . . in later life . . . which may be the independent variables, the independent engines of psychological change in later life" (Hochschild, 1975, p. 559). Therefore, why spin out grand theories? Cruel necessity is all that must realistically be postulated.

Kalish (1972) has proposed limited applicability of disengagement theory to the frail, very old, and terminally ill aged, building upon "the existential necessities" noted by Hochschild (1975).

Of Social Values and the Dying: A Defense of Disengagement

R. A. Kalish

Levels of Disengagement

The author would make two suggestions: First, that the theory of disengagement must be evaluated on three different levels and that each level should be evaluated in terms of whether it refers to psychological disengagement or social disengagement. Further, that the danger of lumping all elderly persons into the same basket is serious—the recently retired, the very old, the terminally ill, each requires a different evaluation, and individual circumstances will influence these crude typologies.

The first of these levels is disengagement as a process, i.e., it occurs. There seems little doubt that disengagement occurs, although the words of some who declare themselves opposed to disengagement suggest that they are trying to eliminate the process by contending that it does not exist. Both psychological and social disengagement undoubtedly do exist. They probably exist in more extreme form for the very old and the dying than for the recently retired. Also, the author would speculate that they are less likely to affect close family relationships than other involvements, and further, that part of that purpose of disengagement is to permit the retention of meaningful family relationships at a relatively undiminished level as long as possible, thus requiring the sacrifice of other kinds of engagement.

The second level is that disengagement is inevitable or, at least, inevitable in this society. Again, the inevitability refers to both psychological and social disengagement, both the retreat from interactions and the retreat from ego-involvements. Here room for disagreement emerges, and many who espouse activity theory in opposition to disengagement theory are really stating that disengagement is not inevitable and, therefore, should not be permitted to occur. An alternative approach would be to accept the need for social disengagement, since energy level and health may require a reduction in social interactions, but deny the necessity of reducing affective involvements. Or, conversely, that reduction of affective involvements should be undertaken to allow greater frequency of more casual interactions. Again, the dying person may be set aside as a unique circumstance, so that both social and psychological disengagement may be inevitable for him, but not for other elderly, since his energy potential may become too limited for more than minimal interaction with close family members. In this regard, there is a need to evaluate his dying trajectory, since a cancer patient is in a different situation than the victim of a heart attack, an accident, or a stroke.

The third level is that disengagement is adaptive. It is this point that produces most of the disagreement. To state that social disengagement is adaptive is to state that reduction in the number and intensity of social interactions can be functional. This may well be acceptable, even to those disliking the concept of disengagement, since it would permit maintaining the more important relationships, most probably with close family members, as long as possible. Social disengagement thus becomes not only inevitable but desirable. Psychological disengagement, on the other hand, suggests reduced richness in life, which can be especially distasteful when other kinds of losses are inevitably occuring. Thus the antidisengagement geriactivist may wish to focus his efforts upon this particular phase of the concept of disengagement: He will disagree with the belief that reduction of affective ties among the elderly (but perhaps not among the terminally ill elderly) is adaptive. Conversely he may work actively toward enabling an elderly person to retain a high level of affective content in his relationships, even though the risk of imminent loss becomes increasingly higher with age. To paraphrase the old gambling adage: Even though it is a game with a high loss probability, it is the only game in town. Nonetheless, when the loss probability is too high, i.e., when death is impending, the game is no longer worth the pain of losing, and disengagement is more readily permitted.

The role of the family in these matters is readily apparent. Thus, if an elderly person has no close family accessible, the process of psychological disengagement may occur with less constraint and may even be seen as more acceptable by geriactivists. Or, if family relationships are hostile and angry, social disengagement may be seen as highly adaptive and, perhaps, inevitable. It is ironic that there are occasions calling for both social and psychological disengagement from family members, where social pressures, guilt, or other factors will not permit it. It is also probable that a family member, or several members, could bring about re-engagement, both psychological and social, in responding to the urgency of the dying person, by overcoming ancient petulance and irritations. It is likely that such re-engagement would be adaptive, even for a terminal patient, although it might produce a compensatory disengagement elsewhere; also, as Kübler-Ross (1969) pointed out, the self-isolation process of the dying person might shortly cause him to disengage from this newly re-established relationship. Other facets of the family relationships of disengaging older persons can be hypothesized.

The personal opinion of the author is that both social and psychological disengagement occur in innumerable older (and many younger) persons; that, given the realities of contemporary society, of the aging process, and of death, both social and psychological disengagement are inevitable, although obviously in varying degrees according to the individual, his intimate relationships—primarily family—and his surrounding; and that both social disengagement and psychological disengagement are adaptive for some persons and under some conditions, but less adaptive or even maladaptive for other persons and situations. When the situation is that of the dying process or imminent death, social disengagement is frequently necessitated by the situation, the individual just not having the energy or the time to remain fully engaged. At this juncture, psychological disengagement would very likely be adaptive in permitting the person to reduce his affect for what he is leaving behind so that the leaving is less painful; nonetheless, it is important to recognize that some persons will find it highly adaptive to be extensively engaged psychologically as long as health and health care permit. (pp. 91–92)

Editor's Conclusion

As this chapter is being written, Jarvick and Russell (1979) have suggested an alternative to disengagement theory. It has been noted that, though low grade chronic anxiety is common in the aged, severe anxiety is infrequently noted. Though the evidence is meager (perhaps because nobody has yet looked for it) it is reasonable to postulate (more reasonable than disengagement) that survival to old age is linked to developing strategies that deal with anxiety by neither of the emergency reactions noted by Selye (1956) and Cannon (1929)—neither the fight nor flight reactions. The optimal reaction when neither fight nor flight is possible is passive acceptance, adaptive flexibility, an increase in introversion; these may be the most appropriate responses to the chronic stresses of aging—a damping of emotions, riding out the storm, playing possum. Apathetic withdrawal, putting mind and emotion in neutral, may be the most adaptive reaction. Those who cannot "disengage" from stress in this manner may be less likely to survive to grow old.

Other theories of aging have been promulgated. Some emphasize differential adjustment by different personality types; Neugarten, et al. (1964), using data of the Kansas City Study of Adult Life, have developed a typology of personalities that adapt differently to the aging process, which is remarkably congruent with the typology conceived by Reichard, et al. (1962). Other broader theories, linking environmental, social, and psychological factors, are not germane to this reader, as these theories have not awakened much controversy in the gerontological community. A summary of these theories may be found in Hendricks and Hendricks (1977, pp. 116–24). They may well prove to be the wave of the gerontological future, but are as yet, by and large, too global to be useful as research models.

Recommended Readings

*Cumming, E. "New Thoughts on the Theory of Disengagement." *International Social Science Journal* 15 (1963):377–393. Also reprinted in R. Kastenbaum, ed., *New Thoughts on Old Age*. New York: Springer, 1964, pp. 53–67.
*———. "Engagement with an Old Theory." *International Journal of Aging and Human Development* 6 (1975):247–51.

Cumming, E. and Henry, W. *Growing Old: the Process of Disengagement*. New York: Basic Books, 1961.

Henry, W. "Engagement and Disengagement: Toward a Theory of Adult Development." In *Contributions to the Psychobiology of Aging*, edited by R. Kastenbaum. New York: Springer, 1965.

*Hochschild, A. "Disengagement Theory: a Critique and Proposal." *American Sociological Review* 40, (1975):553–69.

*Maddox, G. "Disengagement Theory: a Critical Evaluation." *Gerontologist* 9 (1969):80–83.

Streib, G. "Disengagement Theory in Socio-Cultural Perspective. In *New Thoughts on Old Age*, edited by R. Kastenbaum. New York: Springer, 1964, pp. 69–76.

*The major contributions to this chapter's development.

6

On Death and Dying

Death can be beautiful, with this ecstatic guide for dying. $5.
Classified ad in *Harpers Magazine*, October 1978

Editor's Introduction

Death and dying are largely, though of course not exclusively, prerogatives of the elderly. Over half of the deaths occurring are of those over 65. It is not necessary to belabor the point that the upsurge of interest in the matter of death and dying affects the aged more than any other age group. While it may seem perfectly obvious, in this day and age, that death and dying are the province and problem of older pople, it is not at all obvious in historical terms. For most of the existence of mankind on this earth, the average life span was no longer than 25 or 30 years; to have attained an average life span of 70+ is a revolutionary achievement. Those interested in the aged must have an interest in the achievements and shortcomings of thanatology (the study of dying), among whom Dr. Elizabeth Kübler-Ross is best known to the public (1969, 1975).

Her work is too well-known to require elucidation. Everyone knows about her five stages of "growth" in the dying process—from denial through anger, bargaining, and depression to acceptance and peaceful death. Everyone is equally cognizant of her claim for the existence of a heaven of sorts, because some patients resuscitated from cardiac arrest describe their euphoric glimpses of a transcendental world, where often loved ones who preceded them to the great beyond await them with comforting arms. Kübler-Ross has been among the acknowledged pioneers along with Feifel (1959), Kalish (forthcoming), Kastenbaum and Aisenberg (1972), Saunders (1965, 1976), and others who have had the courage to talk about death, not alone to professionals (that was hard enough), but to the dying and their families. She has written sensitively and perceptive-

93

ly on this topic. Unfortunately, the lowering of the taboos on discussing death has brought out a host of ill-prepared advisors, insensitive experts, even charlatans who have oversimplified the complex, difficult, and highly individual task of dying and reduced it to a formula. There are even hospital chaplains whose "counseling" of the dying consists of a brief lecture on the five stages and "Goodbye, you are now ready to die!" Dr. Kübler-Ross is not responsible for these nuts; indeed she is reported to have regretted writing the book as she did (Farber, 1977).

Presented in this section are several issues surrounding death and dying. Dr. Kübler-Ross and others who believe in a life after death have contributed the "out of body" experience as evidence that there is something beyond the grave. Some contrary evidence is offered. Following that is a brief comment by Kalish as to the parallels between Kübler-Ross's concept of the "acceptance" stage of dying and what gerontologists have defined as disengagement.

One of the problems of modern medicine is that it has become so technically proficient that many things can be done. Some of them ought not to be done. There should be a difference in the treatment of the sick and that of the dying. That difference is explicated in the paper by Osmond and Siegler (1976). Some gentle but wise fun is poked at the "death-and-dying people" and their pretensions, for which we acknowledge the contributions of Farber (1977). A physician's perceptions of the problems involved in the "five stages of dying" begins this chapter (Hudson, 1978).

Death, Dying and the Zealous Phase

R. Hudson

Kübler-Ross's conclusions lend themselves to a sort of cookbook approach to dying patients that may be positively harmful in the hands of those armed principally with ardor, the quality that for Bierce characterized "love without knowledge." Here are five stages of dying and a remedy for each. Repressed anger stage? Tear down all the get-well cards or throw a ballpoint pen at the next devil who walks through the door. Depression stage? Merely point out that it is normal to be depressed at the thought of dying, that if you were in their fix, you would be depressed also; besides, take heart, the depressed phase comes just before acceptance, so all will soon be well. It does not matter that the prophetess herself has warned against such simplicities; Freud did the same with psychoanalysis, and two generations of psychiatrists paid scant attention.

We need not belabor the fact that not all patients go lock-stepping through the five stages in identifiable ways. Even if they did, we would not always know how to handle things for every patient apparently wanting our aid. Any given stage can call for widely varying therapeutic approaches. In many instances no one can precisely know what would best serve. A recent personal case speaks to this point. The man (we shall call him Mr. Simon) was a 56-year-old Jewish machinist dying of metastatic carcinoma of the lung. Despite little formal education he was deeply schooled in classic literature and philosophy. (This was never in doubt after the first interview when he asked his visitor if he preferred Ciardi's *Dante* to that of the classical Cary.) His philosophical pursuits had estranged him from the religion of his childhood, and in fact the consultation had been requested precisely because he had made such a forceful case for rational suicide that no one knew quite how to deny his persistent request for a handgun. A social worker had noted that he could not reach the stage of acceptance until he abandoned his cerebral approach in favor of some sort of intuitional revelation. This attitude is attuned to the current emphasis on emotion over intellect and in many instances, perhaps, it would have been proper. In this case, there was good reason to doubt the desirability of such an attack. Every time a probe was made in that direction Mr. Simon promptly returned to rational analysis. Several hours were spent asking what was the sense of it all, agreeing there might be none, seeing that there had to be or life became ridiculous, pursuing the alternatives; if life was indeed ridiculous, deciding that one either reverted to faith or concluded that living itself was the only point of life, and on and on. Early it came out that he was not quite certain that shooting was the best form of suicide. With such obvious ambivalence, this subject was ignored by the consultant and returned to only halfheartedly by Mr. Simon on two later occasions. If he wanted to talk about Socrates and the hemlock, should some therapist insist in saying, "Socrates is well and good, but how do you feel about *your* impending death?" Of course he was denying, but is that always bad? All his adult life he had relied on his rational strengths in attempting to understand events he encountered. Would it have been proper to insist that he approach the even greater riddle of death in a totally different way?

This is not to say that anyone of stature advocates the emotional route as the only way to the acceptance stage of the dying process. It is only to say that a cookbook strategy leads naturally to recipes for managing each stage. The plea is only for the modicum of humility that would have spared medicine so many baneful excesses in the past, the willingness to say, "we don't know yet." We must repeatedly ask ourselves, "Where is it written?" When we do raise the art to something of a science, almost certainly we shall find that the infinite variability of human beings dictates that the cookbook here has no more validity than it does in prescribing digitalis to a patient in heart failure. It is not the zealotry alone that worries, but its association with ignorance under the guise of instant expertise. This does not refer to the honest quacks who quickly infest any area of rapid expansion in medicine. The quacks at least know that they do not know. This may not control their activity but gives them a current cunning about boundaries they may not cross without doing hurt to themselves, which is, of course, their principal concern. The object of concern here is the well-meaning but instant thanatologists now appearing among card-carrying health professionals. One simply cannot read a few books and become proficient in managing the psychology of dying. Bedside training is necessary here just as it is in all clinical medicine. During the zealous phase there will be no certified specialists and of course no standards. The publicizing of the void in terminal psychological care will attract numbers of practitioners limited only by access to patients in a remunerative setting. The potential for damage here is at least as great as it is when any untrained person sets up shop to help others with the emotional problems of living. (pp. 700–701)

Editor's Comment: What about Life after Death?

Kübler-Ross's patients' visions of the hereafter (Taylor and Ingrasci, 1977), and all other arguments for and against life after death, can convince only those who want to be convinced. To the unconvinced, there is no evidence that they are anything other than the euphoria often experienced by those who have miraculously overcome death (one form of the "survivor syndrome"). Death is, by definition, the *end* of the process of dying, when the state is irreversible and any experiences that occur before that end-state "don't cut no ice" with nonbelievers. Indeed, there is "evidence" similar to that of Kübler-

Ross that some resuscitated patients experience having been to hell. According to Dr. Maurice Rawlings (1978), a consultant in advanced life support for the American Heart Association, about half of those resuscitated experience the lovely euphoria described by Kübler-Ross. The other half experience fiery lakes, swarms of creepy, crawly creatures, being taken on conveyor belts to a room full of ovens, and similar terrifying experiences. One might hazard an educated guess that Kübler-Ross is a religious liberal, who believes in some sort of heaven but who cannot belive that the All-Merciful and Loving Parent of us all would establish a real fire-and-brimstone hell. Rawlings, one might suspect, tends toward religious fundamentalism. To at least some extent, patients are attuned to the desires and respond to the cues of the physicians who snatch them from the jaws of death. Patients are likely to tell these demideities whatever they want to hear. Another element to this riddle may be analogous to the behavior of experimental rats in America and Germany. How much of behavior is in the eye of the beholder?

For whatever it is worth, I have "taught" a course in "Death and Dying" that was attended by several nurses who had had experience working in several varieties of intensive care units—myocardial infarct, surgical, and others. None had ever heard of anyone who had ever had a patient describe an experience such as those described by Kübler-Ross or Rawlings. My students note that when a patient begins to talk to a beloved, long-dead relative or friend or describes the beautiful garden with sweet-smelling flowers in which he now finds himself, "you can bet he is slipping fast and you had better call a code (resuscitation) alarm." These "otherworldly" experiences are not found where investigators do not seek them out. Such experiences were not encountered by Massachusetts General Hospital psychiatrists, interviewing patients who survived cardiac arrests. Most of the six survivors described by Hackett (1968) remembered, at most, a dreamlike memory of chest-thumping. Even during the current vogue of "out of body" experiences (Taylor and Ingrasci, 1977), not all investigators characterize the feelings sometimes experienced during life-threatening situations as intimations of immortality, but as an "adaptive, even life-saving, response in many instances. . . . Similar alteration in attention occurs in

marijuana intoxication" (Noyes and Kletti, 1976, p. 26). These investigators characterize the phenomenon as "depersonalization" and
note that mystical phenomena, though part of brief depersonalization experiences of healthy young people, are absent in the desperately ill patients. (This after investigating 114 resuscitations.) Dlin
(1974) also notes a phenomenon of awareness of dying often followed
by acute psychotic reactions, but none of his thirty-five resuscitated
patients report having been in either heaven or hell.

Editor's Introduction: Dying and Disengaging

Kübler-Ross and others noted earlier have accomplished some
admirable tasks. They have lifted the taboo on discussing death and
dying and opened avenues of communication between the living
and the dying. That some have, perhaps unavoidably, gone too far in
the direction of demythologizing and overemphasizing their viewpoints has been considered and will be discussed further. They have
also, perhaps unwittingly, integrated the concept of disengagement
into an area in which it seems to be most appropriate. If those in
terminal stages of chronic illness have less energy to invest in living
and husband these energies by limiting the number and intensity of
relationships and generally loosening the intensity of their ties to
this world, they achieve that neutral emotional state of acceptance,
which pretty well coincides with marked disengagement. Much of
the grieving and mourning process by family members can occur
before death, much as the dying person grieves and mourns his or
her impending departure. Indeed, the freer and open communication being advocated helps to make grief and mourning a family
process, in which they can partake *together*, rather than having the
dying one go through it before his or her death and the others after
it. This mutual process probably occurs naturally in many cases of
terminally ill and older people, whose deaths occur "naturally" after
a period of protracted illness and "on time." This may explain the
concentration of the "death and dying people" on those who "die out
of turn," on deaths of children and young adults. Kübler-Ross makes
this point, which is amplified by Kalish (1972).

Of Social Values and the Dying:
A Defense of Disengagement

R. A. Kalish

"If a patient has had enough time . . . he will reach a stage during which he is neither depressed nor angry about his 'fate.' He will have been able to express his previous feelings, his envy for the living and the healthy, his anger at those who do not have to face their end so soon. He will have mourned the impending loss of so many meaningful people and places and he will contemplate his coming end with a certain degree of quiet expectation. He will be tired and in most cases, quite weak" (1969:99). It is not that Kübler-Ross sees acceptance as a happy stage, but that it is neutral, "almost void of feelings" (1969:100). During this time, the dying person is seen as quite detached, not especially interested in the outside world, and no longer needing much social contact. What Kübler-Ross has described is the disengagement of the dying. She subsequently describes the concern of the family during this period, their difficulty in accepting "that a dying man who has found peace and acceptance in his death will have to separate himself, step by step, from his environment, including his most loved ones" (1969:150). When Cumming and Henry (1961) wrote their original volume on disengagement, the gerontological skies were torn with the anger of retorts that they had far over-extended their interpretation; when Kübler-Ross says very much the same thing, but restricts it to the dying, there seems to be no disagreement voiced. Is it that Kübler-Ross' comments are acceptable or is it that, either by omission or commission, the gerontological community does not encounter her writing or her meaning?

Editor's Introduction: Sickness and Dying

Perhaps part of the problem in dying is that we have confused roles and processes properly involved with illness care with those involved with dying. Behaviors appropriate to reversible illness and its pain and suffering, which involve vigorous therapy and mobilizing the will of the patient to "stick it out," have been extended to the dying. Where in earlier times, death occurred at home in the bosom of the family, deathbed dramatics and all, today death occurs in the hospital, down the corridor furthest from the nursing station, the patient drugged into submission to tubes, needles, and oxygen tents and where, if families do not engage in disruptive behavior, the defeat of medical technology will be all but ignored.

The Dying Role—Its Clinical Importance

H. Osmond and M. Siegler

A hospital chaplain told me this story recently about a man dying of cancer. The battle was ending. Everyone, including surgeon and patient, agreed on that. The patient wanted to go home and die in familiar surroundings. The surgeon refused. "I fought for him for the last eight years and I shall go on till the end," he said. Intimidated by this, the patient died in the hospital, resentful, disgruntled, and wretched. He did not die well or happily.

Some years ago a friend and teacher, Dr. Felix Brown, developed liver cancer. When it became clear that all the good that could be done had been done, he went home to die and his family gathered 'round him. He became steadily weaker, but remained conscious and very cheerful. One day he told his family that he felt very tired, wanted to rest, and would now go to sleep. They came close to him and he died quietly within the hour, thus confounding his colleagues who had predicted that he would be in a coma for about a week. Knowing Felix, we are sure that out-foxing that prediction added some gentle fun to his tranquil departure.

What happened in these two cases? The first man was certainly thought to be dying, for everyone agreed about this. However, because he and his doctor did not recognize that the sick role and the dying role are very different, with separate rights and duties, he died wretchedly, resentful, bitter, thwarted, and ill-disposed toward the same doctor who had fought so hard for his life. Our old friend, who had placed himself firmly in the dying role, died well and the memory of his passing is still recalled lovingly by his family and friends.

What then is the dying role? Medically it can be seen as one of the three exits from the sick role which can be left 1) by recovery, 2) by becoming impaired, and 3) by entering the dying role.

In spite of its immense importance for the practice and teaching of medicine, the sick role, defined by Talcott Parsons (1951), the great Harvard sociologist, has impinged very little on medicine, as any systematic study of medical writing shows. The sick role is governed by Parson's four postulates. These are: 1) exemption from some or all normal responsibilities, 2) blamelessness for the condition—one cannot help being ill or recover by act of will, 3) one is expected to want to get well as soon as possible, and 4) one is expected to seek appropriate help and cooperate with that help. The sick role is highly cross-cultural. It is found in some form in nearly all cultures and also in some animal societies.

Gerald Gordon (1966) discovered the impaired role which, he noted, was so different from the sick role that "in terms of function the two roles are opposite." He stated that "in the case of the impaired role, the social pressure served to aid and maintain normal behavior within the limitations of a given condition, while in the case of the sick role, social pressure serves to discourage normal behavior."

Until recently, the third exit from the sick role has excited little attention, either from doctors or from anyone else. We have so far been unable to find it named anywhere in the literature. We suspect that, like the sick role, the dying role has been so well recognized socially that it has been too familiar either to be perceived clearly or to require definition. In a recent and valuable book, *The Courage to Fail* (Fox and Swaizey, 1974) the distinguished authors do not mention the dying role even though their book discusses at length many problems associated with it. In Van Gennep's classic, *The Rite of Passage* (1960), sickness and dying are strangely absent although pregnancy and funerals are well represented. . . .

We have not yet charted the rights and duties of the dying role to our full satisfaction but our studies already show that, just as Gordon differentiated the sick and the impaired roles, so we can distinguish the sick and dying roles. Take the case of Heidi Biggs. In February 1975 this 14-year-old girl and her mother arrived in Hawaii from their home in Illinois. They were greeted with floral leis and a cake which was inscribed "Heidi, enjoy your trip." Heidi strolled down the main street of Waikiki and then rested before some horseback riding which she anticipated with particular pleasure. The trip was paid for with funds raised by a Canadian who learned that Heidi wanted to see Hawaii before she died. This trip was the last indulgence possible to give her for she died shortly after the plane bringing her home touched down (*Birmingham News*, 1975).

Heidi had a rare untreatable cancer and had only a short time to live. Had her illness been considered treatable, the doctors would have exerted great pressure upon her and her family to come into the hospital and submit to further treatment. They and almost everyone else would have been most critical about her taking a vacation in Hawaii instead of going into a hospital and devoting herself to treatment. Indeed, such an action would have been considered irresponsible and immoral behavior, even though she might have died as soon or sooner in consequence of operations or treatment. However, since she was no longer in the sick role but in the dying role, all sorts of indulgences, like the condemned prisoner's last meal, are countenanced. Among the greatest of these is the right to refuse further treatment.

It may not be the final vacation but the final disposition of the soul which becomes the main consideration for those about to be installed in the dying role. When Samuel Johnson requested his doctor to tell him plainly how things stood with him, the doctor asked whether he thought he could bear the whole truth, whatever it might be. Johnson said that he could and so his doctor told him that without a miracle he would not recover. Johnson remarked "Then I will take no more physic, not even my opiates, for I have prayed that I might render up my soul to God unclouded" (Wain, 1975).

In both the sick role and the dying role, the role holder (the sick or dying person), is given certain concessions by society due to his peculiar state. However, the concessions are not the same, so that if the two roles become confused, the dying person is liable to be damaged and suffer avoidable harm. The line between the sick role and the dying role is not always clear, so that with an increasing number of technical advances in medicine, the possibility of muddle increases. If the doctor fails to concede the dying role when it should be given then an absurd, tragic, and almost obscene mock battle against death occurs in spite of its futility. Some years ago an elderly judge, who had severe cerebral arteriosclerosis and who longed for death, was operated on to renew the battery of his cardiac pacemaker, against his own wishes and those of his wife. He was considered too confused to make this decision and her views were overruled by a court, petitioned by doctors made nervous by the litigious climate of our times. It is unclear whose interests were served by this precaution. They were not, from all accounts, those of the judge or his wife. . . .

During the past sixty or seventy years, medicine has gradually absorbed the dying role, but largely by default. Most doctors would be only too glad to be rid of this unwanted responsibility if only they knew how. It has never been considered a major part of a doctor's role to minister to the dying. His role is to signal that the final act is about to begin and prepare the patient and his family for this event. He sometimes gives a placebo, a harmless and inexpensive medicine, enabling him to maintain a symbolic presence for reassurance. As the doctor withdraws, the main actors in this phase of the drama are ushered in; the family and friends of the dying person, representatives of law, religion, philosophy, and ethics. . . .

Because of the technical achievements made during the recent decades, there is a danger that the last act may become, not a crowning mercy, but a bizarre mixture of science fiction and medico-legal debate.

How did the dying role come to wither away? We believe that this is related to the rise of the modern hospital. It is only during the last fifty to seventy-five years that vast technopalaces have been built for doctors. . . .

The present modern secular hospital reflects the decline of religious authority and the relative rise of Aesculapian (medical) authority. The modern hospital has itself contributed to that decline by providing no appropriate space where the clergy, the family, and the dying person can come together at the time of the impending death. The hospital architecture reflects what is now held to be most important: saving life at any cost. The sick role has squeezed out the dying role, both socially and spatially. Nevertheless, people still die, and many of them die in a hospital. . . .

Some years ago Cicely Saunders (1969) started a hospital called Saint Christopher's where people came to die. Its two chief functions are to ease pain without turning people into vegetables, and to help those who are not going to recover to come to terms with their fate. Dr. Saunders writes, "To go on pressing for acute active treatment at the stage when a patient has gone too far and should not be made to return is not good medicine. There is a difference between prolonging living and what can really only be called prolonging dying. Because something is possible does not mean that it is necessarily either right or kind to do it. One often sees a great weariness with the sort of pain and illness that brings our patients to us, such as that of Sir William Osler who, when he was dying, said, 'I am too far across the river now to want to come back and have it to do all over again.' I do not think he would have given a 'thank you' to someone who pulled him back at that stage. . . ."

How then can we encourage a more realistic approach to death and dying? Perhaps the best way would be for those in the sick role to realize that they have a right to the dying role when they need it, and for them and their relatives to insist they are not deprived of this right should they wish to exercise it. The failure to give the dying role is a recent and mistaken custom which we should now abandon for reasons both of common sense and common humanity. . . .

Such evidence as we possess regarding peri-mortem experience suggests that prolonged and vigorous intrusions into the dying process may convert a peaceful passage to oblivion or some other state of being into hellish torment. The Gestapo used repeated part-drowning followed by resuscitation as an exquisite torture; it was not expected that the procedure would help the resuscitated.

Surely medicine, which has done so much to make life better for so many people, should turn its attention to assuring that, when the time comes, the dying role will be made available to those who require it. Medicine must not intrude upon the final hours of those who no longer need its services, however well-intentioned such intrusions may be. . . .

It is not always easy to tell people that they are dying and many of us hesitate to do so, but the evidence suggests that false reassurances, however well-intended, do much more harm than good. Freud (Roazen, 1975) turned with "blazing eyes" upon his trusted physician and friend, Felix Deutsch, who had, with the agreement of other psychoanalysts, concealed from him the seriousness of his cancer. "By what right?" Freud asked him in fury. Deutsch could not answer this and Freud never again trusted him fully, although he was fond of him. Our patients may well ask us by what right we deny them that universal last refuge—the dying role. . . .

Today we can prolong the sick role, sometimes almost indefinitely, but we may do this to the detriment of the patient whose interest may be submerged in technical virtuosity. It is our duty to be vigilant, not only to relieve our patient's suffering, but to insure that when the time comes they have an easy and graceful access to the dying role. One day we ourselves will require the same watchful help so that, "the last act crowns *our* play."

Editor's Comment: Some Excesses in the Study of Death and Dying

Whenever social changes occur, particularly in deeply rooted values and especially when taboos are violated, the pendulum generally swings too far. Profundity degenerates into rhetoric, no matter how pretty; the insensitivity of the new is as unfortunate as the old, only in the opposite direction. Farber (1977) illustrates some of the excesses that can, have, and still do occur in the field of thanatology, the study of dying and death.

Farber presents a lovely ironic "put down" of the let's-teach-everyone-about-death-and-dying school of thanatologists. We attempt here a summary of some major points, but refer readers to the heartily recommended original paper.

Some thanatalogical enthusiasts seem to have the idea that—as in any other "ology"—they can arrive at prediction and control of the subject matter under investigation. Death can be studied and tamed; that devilment can be put in a bottle, whence it can be dissected, analyzed, and made ordinary. We can learn to "accept" death, to remove its anguish and terror and make it commonplace—

just another part of the life cycle, though of course of some obvious importance. Now, while death may be a problem of some intensity to some of us at one time or another, not all problems necessarily have solutions. Some aspects of life are unfathomable. See, for example, Farber's (1964) discussion of sex. Freud, Kinsey, and Masters and Johnson have demystified sex and the thanatologists want to do the same with death. There is one major difficulty: not much can be done about death, but perhaps something can be done about dying and fear of death. Farber doubts (as we do) that death is an ever-present fear to too many of us. Some in the grip of guilt of an unworthy life (see the Russian Lord bemoaning his wicked life in Jacob Wasserman's *The World's Illusion*, 1976) may be awed and appalled at the irreversibility of their wretchedness. Others encounter brushes with death in moments of major accidents, experienced or avoided by a bit of good fortune, or of life-threatening illness. There are moments when one realizes how infinitely precious are the ordinary events of our humdrum lives, moments that Thornton Wilder celebrates in his play *Our Town* (1938), which has been performed by almost every high school drama group since it was written. But most of us slip in and out of awareness of the looming presence. Why on earth must we be constantly drilled into a desensitization to death (which somehow, at the same time, makes us celebrate the preciousness of every moment)? One may suppose that almost any moment of our lives (except perhaps when we are in terminal stages of cancer or emphysema) is better than nothingness, if we must make that comparison; but why must we? Who needs it, not younger people at the beginning of their adult lives, nor mature people who at last think they are beginning to know what life is all about? A life cannot be lived as though every moment was a peak of precious gold. We need some valleys of relaxation, of ordinariness in each day. There are also times when we do not, or cannot, wring the ultimate sweetness out of every moment. Disappointment, unhappiness, failure, even monotony are part of life. These less than ecstatic experiences are not preparations for death as some thanatologists preach. It is simply untrue that "Everytime one says goodbye, he dies a little," because the last good-bye is the *last* (at least in this existence) and is, therefore, not comparable to any other. Most of life is not preparation for death; to the contrary, we rightly concentrate on the daily process of living, with its own cycles and rhythms. Again, why dwell on the end? It will come when it comes. We know it must come; in between the beginning and the end, we live, in varying, ever-changing degrees of awareness of the end.

Farber presents some wryly amusing examples of thanatological zealotry (to use Hudson's term, presented earlier). It is regrettable that space considerations prohibit reproduction of his entire paper; this should not prevent readers from proceeding to the nearest library and enjoying Farber's humanistic, commonsense, and totally delightful contribution to the literature on death and dying.

Death is the end of life; it may be the beginning of something that we can only imagine and hope for. Death must never become the be-all and end-all of life, but just the end, however mysterious and awesome.

Recommended Readings

Farber, L. "O death, Where is Thy Sting-a-ling-a-ling?" *Commentary* 63 (November 1977):35–43.

Feifel, H., ed. *The Meaning of Death*. New York: McGraw-Hill, 1959.

Kalish, R. *Death, the Process of Dying and Grief*. Monterey, Calif.: Brooks/Cole, forthcoming.

Kastenbaum, R. and Aisenberg, R. *The Psychology of Death*. New York: Springer, 1972.

Kübler-Ross, E. *On Death and Dying*. New York and London: Macmillan, 1969.

Weisman, A. *On Dying and Denying: A Psychiatric Study of Terminality*. New York: Behavioral Publications, 1972.

Part Four

Cultural and Social Dimensions

7

Aging: A More Difficult Problem for Women Than for Men?

If particular care and attention is not paid to the ladies, we are determined to foment a rebellion and we will not hold ourselves bound by any laws in which we have had no voice or representation.

Letter of Abigail Adams to her husband John Adams, 1774.

Editor's Introduction

Allied to the problem of disengagement is the possibility of differential aging process for the two sexes. It has been more or less assumed that, since males presumably have a greater attachment to work roles, their problems in disengaging (or at least in finding satisfactions alternate to work) would be greater than that of females. We present here three papers that argue:

1. Yes, males and females are different, but as women are changing, they will lose their "feminine" passivity and become increasingly activist—and good for them! (Cora Martin).

2. Yes, males and females are different, and discontinuity built into the feminine role (that is, the changes from work to motherhood—often more than once—to work that is often marginal to their lives, not "a career") makes females more flexible and less rigidly structured, and makes feminine adjustment to aging easier (Chrysee Kline).

3. Females, being the powerless, suppressed half of the world, have a harder time in aging, but male gerontologists have ignored their problems (Diane Beeson).

Lavender Rose or Gray Panther?

C. Martin

Lavender Rose or Gray Panther? The title is designed to call attention to two extremes of life styles that characterize the older woman.

You see, we need different kinds of programs and services for roses and panthers. And if we are going to be planners, preparing for the aged in our society, we need to know something about who the aged are, who they will be, and how they get to be the way they are.

We can already make good predictions about the older people of 2000 or 2010 because we already know a lot about them. They will be largely women. If we look at the way women have been (and are being) socialized we might get some clues as to the kinds of programs they will need.

First, let us look at the process of socialization as it has affected the women who are "old" today. By socialization I mean the process by which we learn to act so that people around us approve of our behavior because we live up to society's expectations. They say, "You are a nice woman" not, "You are an aggressive female."

Socialization continues throughout the life cycle. We are continually learning new roles. But early socialization is very important and, since our culture is more or less consistent, it reinforces the lessons of childhood with expectations for similar behavior later. For example, society taught little girls in the early 1900's to be nice, obedient, quiet little girls. In the 1920's, they were expected to be respectable married women, devoting their energies to having contented husbands and well-behaved children. In the 70's we expect them to be nice old ladies. We have created, in this age group, a garden of lavender roses.

Of course, not all have thus bloomed. There were, after all, the flappers of the 20's. But most of them settled down in the 30's and followed the pattern. These older women often have a very hard time as widows (which most are by this time), dealing with the impersonal social system which characterizes today's society. They always had a father, or a husband, or at least a brother or son to buffer them from the outside world. But now they don't. They must cope alone with an impersonal system which often terrifies them and of which they are suspicious.

My friends working for social security tell me that they often find widows who have never written a check, who have no idea of how much money was in the estate, who know nothing about money management. They are vulnerable to fraud and do not know what benefits are due them.

They are suspicious of "government" and tend to see any benefits as a handout. Will older women always be this vulnerable?

I think the answer is a resounding no, but I'm not sure when we can expect the change from more roses to more panthers.

Let us briefly examine the traditional role of women in our society and how it is changing.

Traditionally we have expected girls to be gentle, nonaggressive, noncompetitive, dependent, and emotional. Girls are sent to school but it is made clear to them that their main purpose in life is to be a wife and mother. Jobs are necessary but they are never primary. They serve to make some money before marriage for a big wedding; perhaps, after marriage in the early years to help accumulate enough capital to buy a new house, or to put a husband through school; then there is a period of "nesting." When the last child goes to school, the wife/mother often returns to the labor force to make "extra" money for the needs—or luxuries—of the family, to send children through college, etc. Finally comes retirement. But even retirement for women has usually been adjusted so that they can leave the labor force earlier than men (at reduced retirement benefits, of course) thus retiring at the same time as their husbands. Even the end of their working career is tied to their husband's departure from the work force, not their own ability or desire to continue to make a contribution.

Some excerpts from a widely used psychology text prove the point. In *Adulthood and Aging,* Douglas Kimmel (1974) describes the personality development of women:

> Because of women's investment in the marriage relationship, because of their history of assessing themselves by others' responses, and because they really do perceive reality in interpersonal terms, they overwhelmingly define and evaluate identity and femininity within the context of marriage. . . . (p. 166)
>
> Passivity in the sense of indrawing, or evolving a rich, empathic, intuitive inner life—in contrast to activity directed outward—may be a necessary part of the personality equipment of healthy women. . . . Certainly not all women are passive and not all men are aggressive; but at this point in time in our society these characteristics seem to stand out as differential aspects of femininity and masculinity. (p. 164)

Kimmel seems to say not only that this is the state of affairs but that it is the preferred state: It is "healthy." What will happen when these dependent, "healthy" women are widowed?

Another author, while supporting the point of view that these qual-

ities are expected of women, questions whether or not they are "healthy."
He says:

> The cost in terms of always having to assume a dependent, secondary
> role is most telling on some women. To assume some responsibility, to assert
> their independence, to respond aggressively to a problem are all unfeminine
> and interpreted as attempts to challenge the male's authority. Woman's role
> becomes that of an object to be admired and used by men; she is there to
> meet his needs as mistress, mother, and housekeeper. If she questions this
> role and challenges the limits placed upon her, she is demeaned, ridiculed,
> and if perchance successful, immediately defined as "not a real woman."
> (McKinney, 1976, p. 138)

These expectations of what women should be are being presented to
college students today. They are certainly descriptive of those 80+ today.
Their needs are financial management training, protective services, and
"helping" programs of various kinds.

But the winds of change are blowing, if not always through psychology
texts. Cartoonists are more attuned to the times than some psychologists!
One of my favorite strips is *Peanuts*. In one, Lucy, reading a composition to
her class says:

> And so World War II came to an end. My grandmother left her job in the
> defense plant and went to work for the telephone company. We need to study
> the lives of great women like my grandmother. Talk to your own grand-
> mother today. Ask her questions. You'll find she knows more than peanut
> butter cookies! Thank you!

My generation has had much of the same childhood socialization as
our mothers but it was attenuated by the social upheaval of the great
depression. Then WWII encouraged women to leave the household and
join the labor force. And, though there was a mass exodus by most women
from that force as the war ended, in 1974, 53 percent of women between
45–54 were working. Most of us were or had been married (more than 90
percent) yet, increasingly, we find ourselves at midlife living in one-person
households. We are learning independence. We, the middle-aged group,
are less ruled by the traditional concept of the women's place, yet we have
not moved as far as many have supposed. We still value the traditional
womanly virtues and are reluctant to appear aggressive or competitive—
despite the "assertive" training of the more liberal feminists among us. Of
course, this has some good payoffs. We have fewer heart attacks and other
stress-related illnesses than our male counterparts and live longer.

As we, the coming generation of aged, arrive on the scene, our first needs are not likely to be for the mastery of the rudiments of financial management or protective agencies. We probably will need to be taught the rudiments of political activism. Robert Butler points out "There is a sturdy and hopefully growing group of old women who are undaunted and look to life with enthusiasm. Old women will not accept their bleak lot forever because they have the brains, money, and voting strength to do something about it." So planners for programs for the aged for the years 2000+, look alive! You are going to have to adjust your planning for us. Gray Panthers, here we come!

The Socialization Process of Women: Implications for a Theory of Successful Aging

C. Kline

Literature dealing with the occupational involvement of Americans has for the most part been based on male work history, and, except for very recent working generations, neglects the substantially different pattern of women (see, for example, Hughes, 1958; de Grazia, 1964; Kreps, 1971). Jackson (1971) has commented that this reflects "an implicit assumption that the working roles of women are relatively unimportant and that retirement is not a significant stage for women."

Career Development

. . . [The modal older widow today, as seen by Lopata and Steinhart (1971)] had a very uneven employment history and had dropped out of the labor market several times during her life, withdrawing to the home to perform the roles of wife, mother, and housewife. In general, however, the work histories of these older women reflect frequent engagement in the work world. Most of those respondents who had continuous or almost continuous work histories shared several characteristics: they spent relatively few years in marriage, entering late in life and/or being widowed or separated; they had no children or only one offspring; and they moved around frequently. The jobs they took were the ones available conveniently at the time they were looking, with no program of career-type succession. Part-time work was common after retirement.

Despite the heavy use of the working world during their life cycle, the older women interviewed in Chicago did not place much value on the role of worker in the list of social roles most often performed by women. The role of worker is not assigned major importance by widows, women who never married, and those who never performed the role of mother. The American culture, locating women in the home as wives and mothers, has had so strong an influence on housewives (Lopata, 1971a) and widows (Lopata, 1972) as to prevent the roles of worker, citizen, and even friend from reaching the top three positions in a six-rank scale of importance.

Roles

. . . Each person normally has several roles to enact because of the various positions occupied in the different institutional aspects of the social structure. In the context of role theory, the enactment of these multiple roles is considered to be the primary basis for most of a person's behavior, attitudes, values, prestige, and personal integration. . . .

The problem of analyzing roles at any stage of the life cycle is complicated by the fact that the person has a number of intersecting and overlapping roles which must be undertaken—sometimes simultaneously and sometimes sequentially, according to the expectations of that particular situation. This problem is accentuated for the female who, according to Atchley (1972), is under greater pressure to assume a number of conflicting roles throughout the life cycle than is the male. For the female, the various roles of worker, housewife, and mother occupy different priority positions at different points throughout the life cycle. Although the male's "role set," or "complement of role specializations" (Biddle and Thomas, 1966) throughout the life cycle also typically consists of a number of roles, the role of worker consistently occupies the greatest area of "role space."

The reasons for the predominance of the role of worker are twofold: (1) it is the one role which most frequently takes precedence over other roles, and (2) the one which derives greater societal rewards relative to rewards from other male roles (Palmore, 1965).

Work role. . . . The employment figures of women in the labor force often camouflage a minimal level of involvement. Only 42% of those women who worked some time in 1967 did so full time the year round (Women's Bureau, 1969). Thus, despite a seeming gradual change in attitude of the traditional culture toward women's roles, the intermittent nature of the female work career will most likely continue, and the work cycles of women will remain clearly distinguishable from those of men.

Lopata (1966) maintains that the social role of housewife has a unique cycle compared to other roles, involving relatively little anticipatory socialization, very brief time devoted to the "becoming" stage, and a rather compressed and early peak. It can be performed during the major part of the life cycle of a woman, yet "its entrance, modifications, and cessation are usually not a consequence of its own characteristics of rhythm but of those other roles." She goes on to explain that some women never become "inside-located," so that the return to work or other community involvement (of married women) after the birth of the children is rapid and complete. Women who have placed themselves in the home and for whom the housewife role became important may be attracted to the outside or forced out of the inside by a feeling of obligation to help in the financial support of the family, or through crises such as widowhood. Those who do not go out completely, but do so part time, include women who have never cut off ties with the outside, or who develop new lines of connection. They most frequently combine both orientations through the addition of some outside role, such as part-time worker, without letting such identification grow into a total commitment. Most of the aforementioned Chicago interviewees, even those who had full time employment outside of the home, expressed an "inside" identity.

Housewife role. The "shrinking circle" stage in the social role of housewife starts when the first child is married or has left home and is very difficult for women who have invested their lives in that role and who do not have alternative sources for the focusing of identity. According to Lopata (1966), the "shrinking" of the "circle" removes many of the sources of prestige without any choice or control on the part of the woman whose identity is bound with it. No matter how well she performs it, how many and how important are the persons for whom it is performed, or how significant is the role in the lives of recipients, modern society automatically decreases the ability of the role of housewife to serve as a center of relations. Thus, "the housewife ceases to perform the role at a high plateau level, long before capacity to carry out its duties decreases, providing a reason or excuse for its cessation." Changes in the role come basically and primarily from changes in characteristics of the circle prior to any changes in her which could provide justification for decreasing functionality. Furthermore, the shrinking of the role importance of housewife and mother cannot always lead to a shift of self and of role-focus to a concentration on the role of wife, if such an emphasis was absent, since the husband tends still to be highly involved in the role of worker.

Also, according to Lopata (1966), for those aging women who have survived the "shrinking circle" stage, fewer decision-making problems, a lack of pressure from demanding and often conflicting roles, satisfaction with past performance of the role of housewife and with the products of the role of mother, and prior adjustment to the lack of centrality in the lives of children can all contribute to a relatively high degree of satisfaction in the later years. For those who are not widows, the focal nature of the role of wife may be increased with the retirement, or "fade out," from occupational roles on the part of the spouse. Widowhood is more likely to occur for females than for males (Lopata, 1972); at any point during the life cycle, death of a spouse could cause a major transformation in the social role of housewife and could demand a role realignment. . . .

Retirement role. The facts *are*, however, that the female is constantly undergoing modifications in the characteristics of each assigned role as she enters different stages of the life cycle or changes her definition of the role, in response to events external to the person. Heyman (1970) remarks that while some wives may retire as many as three different times during a lifetime, these retirements obviously differ from the "retirement" of a man who at a relatively advanced age and with declining physical health is facing a single, final separation from his central life role as a wage-earner and principal provider for his family. The male is faced with loss of what has heretofore been conceived as a permanent work role, reduced economic resources, and necessity for role realignment and the need for new role opportunities. For today's elderly women, on the other hand, retirement may have begun quite early in her lifetime and have recurred periodically.

There currently exists considerable disagreement as to the impact of retirement upon the male. Miller's (1965) identity crisis theory suggests that retirement in and of itself negatively influences the quality of one's life, while Atchley's (1971) identity continuity theory posits that work is not necessarily at the top of several roles on which one's identity rests and that its removal is not regarded negatively by most retired people. However, there is a general consensus in the literature that retirement rarely poses any problems for women because "she is merely giving up a secondary role in favor of the primary roles of housewife, mother, and grandmother" (Palmore, 1965).

Role continuity and discontinuity. . . . [I]t appears that the impact of socialization on American women creates *impermanence* in the form of role loss and repeated adjustment to change in the life situation—and that this socialization process facilitates adjustment of women to old age.

Our society defines "permanence" as having a long-lasting, viable social and economic role. While it appears that this "permanence" is relatively accessible to at least middle-majority males, for women it is tenuous and thwarted. Women of all educational, geographical, and economic positions have been subjected to changes produced by our modern industrial society. Increasing mobility, for example, has changed the complexion of American society in the diminution of the extended family structure in its varied form as well as its demands upon individuals. The striving of women for permanence is dead-ended numerous times during the life cycle, resulting in role discontinuity or change in life situation. This striving for permanence is periodically redirected until old age when societal roles for the aged, both male and female, are further withdrawn.

Failure to attain permanence is exhibited throughout the entire social life cycle of women. Role losses impede attaining permanence before facing the impermanence impact of old age. Symbols of permanence that are thwarted, resulting in role discontinuity and changes in life situation are numerous.

As stated by Steinman (1963), the feminine role is not only ill-defined, but full of contradictions, ambiguities, and inconsistencies. Education, for instance, prepared women for membership in the labor force; yet many parents still raise their daughters with a view of marriage rather than furthering their personal development through employment. The women who are processed through the educational system and then marry experience a strong role discontinuity, as described by Decter (1971). For the woman who disbands her work role to give priority to roles of mother and housewife, there is discontinuity when the children leave home or become increasingly independent of home and parents. Another role discontinuity to consider is the disrupted marital status such as widowhood. In 1968, the wife was the surviving spouse in 70% of all marriages broken by the death of one partner (Lopata, 1971b). Although men also suffer the loss of husband role through widowhood, the loss is experienced by fewer numbers of men and is not coupled with financial loss due to widowhood.

Thus, role discontinuity and change in life situation are more likely suffered by women than men. Adjustments to the discontinuities are imposed on women by society through the socialization process.

It is suggested here, then, that precisely because women *are* subjected to repeated role discontinuities and changes in life situation to which they adjust, the final adjustment to old age is made more easily by them.

Readjustment Theory

Cottrell (1942) maintains that an individual will make a facile adjustment to a role change to the extent that he has undergone anticipatory preparation for that role situation. Women have had considerable experience in adjusting to age-linked changes (children leaving home, meno-

pause) and have therefore become accustomed to change and impermanence. Thus, women are not as devastated as men are likely to be when old
age, another impermanence, separates them from the productive, involved, financially independent world of middle age; and the adoption of
new roles and the giving up of middle-age roles should be relatively more
facile for women than for men. If this theory of repeated readjustment
fosters adjustment to old age for women more readily than for men is valid,
one should be able to demonstrate that the process of adjustment to aging,
especially as it reflects a response to impermanence or discontinuity, is
different for men than for women.

Mulvey (1963) organized what data she had found on characteristics of
women's vocational behavior into seven career patterns, defined in terms
of a career with and without marriage, and with and without work. Her
study of women between the ages of 50 and 60 years concludes that high life
satisfaction is associated with career patterns marked by: (1) return to
career after children entered school ("interrupted-work primary"), (2) entry upon deferred career ("delayed-work secondary"), (3) contribution of
talent and time to volunteer activities when children were young ("stable
homemaking-work secondary"), (4) continuous and simultaneous home-
making and working. The vocational behavior of women who displayed the
least degree of life satisfaction was characterized by a single, continuous
role of either homemaker or worker over the adult life-span. The woman
with a greater degree of life satisfaction has experienced more discontinuity
and change of primary roles over the lifetime.

Dunkle (1972) reanalyzed data from Schooler's (1969) study of noninstitutionalized elderly to investigate the relationship of length of time at
residential location, distance moved, change in marital status, and changes
in position within the labor force to morale in old age. The value of her work
in application to this paper's hypothesis is greatly enhanced by the inclusion of sex differentiation in her sample. Her results show that 47.1% of the
men experiencing only a small degree of change in residence, marital
status, and work involvement have high morale, while 51.8% of those men
who have experienced a considerable amount of change over the life cycle
display high morale, a difference of 4.3 percentage points; 6.3% more
women who display a large amount of change over their lives have higher
morale than the women characterized by stability in residence, marital
status, and work involvement. Furthermore, Dunkle's data show that
almost twice as many women as men experience change with relation to the
tested variables.

With admittedly weak measures in the sense that the data were not
originally intended for this purpose, Dunkle's study suggests that women

are socialized differently from men such that they were in the past more likely to experience discontinuity and impermanence, and that women, in fact, are better able to adjust in old age as a result of this past impermanence in life situations. It seems, therefore, that if discontinuity could be shown to be positively associated with adjustment to old age as measured by morale, there would be important implications for a theory of successful aging, based on discontinuity and impermanence over the life cycle.

Work and Leisure Patterns

. . . Little is known about people's perceptions of the worth of free time; certainly, there is no evidence of the price that will be paid for time off. Most important, there is the question of whether leisure becomes more or less valuable as one grows older. Research might indicate that retirement in the optional years has the effect of conferring leisure on man when he least wants it—a curious inversion of the notion that youth is wasted on the young. The total number of workers involved in career changes during middle age or later worklife might increase, moreover, if such changes were made to be viable alternatives to present continuous cycles of employment.

Senator Mondale (U.S. Congress, Senate, Special Committee on Aging, 1969), a member of the Senate Special Committee on Aging, called for the altering of traditional work lifetime patterns, including institution of sabbaticals, phased retirement, trial retirement, and part-time work arrangements for those near retirement years. Such experiments, however, have been limited. For most elderly males, retirement, whether compulsory or voluntary, has provided the first opportunity for considerable amounts of leisure time throughout all of the adult years. It is no wonder then that renouncing the primary work role and substituting new roles for which there has been little chance for "rehearsal" presents difficulties for the male.

Lopata and Steinhart (1971) suggest it might be valuable for our society to assume that few persons actually benefit from working in one occupation for more than perhaps ten years, and that, with some exceptions, those who do produce diminishing returns for the organization. More efficient methods of education could then be introduced to retrain people at the end of each "natural cycle" of involvement in a particular occupation. We still lack adequate re-engagement procedures in the work world, because of a myth that modern workers work continuously and have steady careers from education to retirement. This fiction does not reflect lives of men, let alone women.

Career Flexibility

Recently, important strides are beginning to be made in liberating women to engage in meaningful employment in liberating society at large to make positions of power available to women. Perhaps the seeming goal to attain the same rigid, life-long role to which most males in our society are now subjected should be reconsidered by women's activist groups. If the theory that impermanence and discontinuity over the adult life cycle exert a direct effect upon positive adjustment to old age is valid, then a new system of career flexibility should be adopted as the new battle cry by men and women alike.

Women in Aging Studies: A Critique and Suggestions*

D. Beeson

Social gerontology, following similar trends in other social sciences, is giving increasing attention to female subjects. This is an appropriate development since gerontology, like other social sciences, has tended to focus predominately on male subjects (Birren et al., 1963:7; Holmes and Jorgensen, 1971). In order to suggest directions for research on aging women, this paper will critically examine the treatment of women in some important studies.

I will show that when women have been included as subjects their experience of aging has frequently been compared to that of men and evaluated as less problematic, less traumatic, and their difficulties seen as more easily resolved. This view contrasts sharply with nonacademic writings on aging. I will show that the discrepancy is related to theoretical and methodological assumptions, and propose an approach which is essential if social gerontologists are to fill the gaps now extant in the field.

*The research for this paper was partially supported by NIH Training Grant No. HD 00238 from the National Institute of Child Health and Human Development. The author gratefully acknowledges her special debt to Carroll Estes for her assistance in the formative stages of this paper, and to Virginia Olesen and Fred Davis for their encouragement in this effort.

Evaluations of Aging as Experienced by Men and Women

Retirement is seen by many gerontologists as "the most crucial life change requiring a major adjustment of the older person" (Atchley, 1972:103). However, such evaluations actually refer only to male persons, as Atchley (1972:105) clarifies by adding, "Although most women have had work experience, their orientation to work is apparently not strong enough to cause any significant problems in retirement."

Retirement has received more attention than any other issue related to later life because of assumptions about its salience for men. Women who retire have been neglected because of parallel assumptions about the relative unimportance of work in their lives. Such a position is made explicit in the work of Cumming and Henry (1961), authors of disengagement theory, who on the basis of thirty-six working women in their Kansas City sample concluded:

> Retirement is not an important problem for women because . . . working seems to make little difference to them. It is as though they add work to their lives the way they would add a club membership (Cumming and Henry, 1961:144).

Although their sample included twenty unmarried women they further concluded that work

> does not express the whole woman in the way that work no matter how uncongenial tends to express the whole man. . . . The basic division of labor between men and women assigns to the woman the task of sociability, of keeping the social system she belongs to free of tension, of maintaining the system's integrity against disruptive inner disturbances (Cumming and Henry, 1961:144).

Twelve years later, Zena Blau states her similar evaluation in this way:

> Retirement . . . deprives a man of the respect accorded the breadwinner in the American family and constrains him to assume a role similar to that of a woman. In this respect, retirement is a more demoralizing experience for men than for women. Women may choose to work, but according to cultural prescription they are not obliged to do so (Blau, 1973:29).

. . . Assumptions of this nature have been so powerful that they have rarely been tested directly, yet evidence which challenges them is beginning to emerge. For example in 1967 Lowenthal, Berkman, and Associates found in their San Francisco study that retired women were more likely to be psychiatrically impaired than retired men.

In a recent report of one of the few longitudinal studies of retirement, and one of the few studies of retirement to include women respondents, Streib and Schneider (1971) came to two conclusions which challenge previous assumptions and findings of gerontologists. First, they concluded that retirement does not have the "broad negative consequences for the older person" that they had expected (Streib and Schneider, 1971:163) (In this case they are actually referring to male persons). They found a "more positive set of consequences than had been hypothesized." Second, they reported

> more surprising is the fact that women who retire report a sharper increase in feelings of uselessness than do their retired male counterparts. This finding certainly suggests that further research is needed to examine the stereotyped idea that the male retiree will find it harder to occupy his time than the older woman who retires (Streib and Schneider, 1971:161).

It is clear that assumptions by gerontologists which dismiss problems of women and overestimate the problematic nature of the male experience have existed and still persist around the issue of retirement.

The major transition of the aging woman has long been considered to be widowhood. Let us briefly examine the assumptions and conclusions about the significance of this experience. One cannot help but notice the common practice among gerontologists of comparing widowhood for women to retirement for men. The purpose of such a comparison is not clear, but the conclusion is invariably one which dismisses widowhood for women as less significant than retirement for men. Remarkably, widowhood is sometimes even evaluated as a welcome transition, while again emphasizing the traumatic nature of the so-called male equivalent—retirement.

Cumming and Henry (1961:156) argue in comparing widowhood for women to retirement for men:

> On the whole, resolutions of these problems of disengagement are much easier for women than for men. . . . Integrating herself into both the larger society and small social systems without a husband is a problem, but a relatively easy one for a widow. In the first place, widowhood is an honored state. . . . Finally, widows have a ready-made made peer group and there is reason to believe that they join this very happily. There is, in fact, some evidence in our interviews of considerable frustration among some married

women over being *unable* to join the society of widows, a frustration especially true of wives of retired husbands.

Generally, disengagement theorists argue that women have a "smoother
passage" made possible apparently because aging for them begins earlier
and lasts longer.

Similar assumptions remain dominant in current work. In 1973 Zena
Blau writes:

> Though widowhood, like retirement, signifies the involuntary loss of a
> significant role, it does not have the invidious implications for the social
> position of older people that retirement does. . . . Retirement threatens the
> individual's self-esteem, whereas no similar threat is inherent in widowhood.
> Retirement, more so than widowhood, lessens opportunities for daily social
> contacts and is therefore more demoralizing (Blau, 1973:32).

Moving even further along the theoretical spectrum from functional-
ism, Cavan (1962) has also felt it necessary to compare the aging experiences of men and women and concluded that widowhood is recognized to
be a severely disturbing transition, but for the widow in contrast to the
retiring male she finds that the culture has devised several appropriate
self-images including the grandparent role which is essentially a maternal
one and therefore presents more difficulty for the grandfather.

Even loss of a spouse is considered most devastating when the surviving partner is male. Cumming and Henry (1961:160), for example, argue
that women are better able than men to establish "quasi-relationships" and

> better able to live alone because they are in command of the necessary
> domestic skills and it is appropriate for them to exercise them. This is not so
> for men; even when they are good at housework, they are ashamed of it.

Thus we have numerous judgments of the woman's experience as
"smoother," "less demoralizing" and "easier." There is little or no empirical
basis for these conclusions. The justification in each case is essentially
theoretical. Some form of role theory provides the basis for each evaluation.

Another View

Students of aging cannot help but be struck by the contrast between
journalistic and scholarly accounts of the female experience of aging. Susan
Sontag's (1972) article, "The Double Standard of Aging," powerfully docu-

ments how cultural differences work to the disadvantage of women. Lynn Caine's (1974) book *Widow* describes her own experience of widowhood in terms of grief, loneliness, financial problems, and changes in self-conception bearing little resemblance to social-psychological insights offered in gerontological literature.

Readers of women's publications find articles that emphasize economic and social-psychological problems and issues that are rarely mentioned in gerontological literature. These articles include discussions of inequities in social security legislation. Major complaints are that homemakers receive no benefits for their own work. They qualify as dependents only after twenty years of marriage to the same man [recently lowered to ten years—HJW]. Widows under 60 without dependent children receive no benefits (Ahern, 1974). Another major problem of older women, noted by Berquist (1973), is re-entry into the paid labor force after years as homemakers. Sex discrimination is compounded by age discrimination and she argues that confidence is usually low even where older women have credentials that are adequate or better than those of competing males.

Social gerontologists have contributed very little to the understanding of the universal phenomenon of female menopause. Neugarten's (Neugarten et al., 1963) work raised interesting questions about differences in the meaning of menopause for older and younger women. Bart's work (1971) elaborated on the social elements in depression among middle-aged women which may contribute to or be confused with symptoms of menopause. Yet such issues are little researched and more attention has probably been given the question of whether or not there is such a thing as "male menopause." In an effort to understand their experience older women are now turning to each other, rather than to the experts, by forming "menopause rap groups."

A double standard of physical attractiveness that creates anxiety in women decades before it is an issue for men has also received attention (Brabec, 1974) in popular women's publications. The absence of attention to many of these issues in gerontological literature has been observed by the Coordinator of the Task Force on Older Women of the National Organization of Women (Sommers, 1974). As a partial explanation she has suggested the tendency of our culture to be more concerned with "those who rise and fall, than those who never rise at all."

One might be tempted to explain the discrepancy between the issues addressed in non-academic writings and those recognized in gerontological literature as the difference between propaganda and scholarship. The difficulty with this explanation is that special problems of older women such as greater poverty (Butler and Lewis, 1973:90), increased prevalence of living alone and higher incidence of institutionalization (Brotman, 1974:250), disadvantage for remarriage (Butler and Lewis, 1973:91), and even symbolic denigration (Arnoff, 1974) are confirmed by statistical and demographic evidence. Somehow these differences do not show up in theoretical statements, nor do they often lead to generalizations by scholars about the situation of aging women.

Conscious discrimination against women by scholars, particularly in a field where women have been active, is not an adequate explanation. Theoretical and methodological styles have worked to perpetuate dominant culture values even where women have received attention. These values may accurately be labeled as sexist or andro-centrist. Theoretical and methodological fashions which facilitate these values or at least fail to expose them must be recognized if we are to avoid sexism in research.

Theoretical and Methodological Issues

. . . Studies, particularly in survey research, which have perpetuated the emphasis on the aging male by revealing the subtleties and difficulties of his problems while remaining unresponsive to problems of older women are studies where the categories of experience to be investigated have been predefined by the researchers. This structuring of the problem has the effect of preventing definitions of reality other than those anticipated by the researcher from emerging clearly and fully, even in empirical work. Mueller (1970) points out that the predefinitions which form the standard political language assure maintenance of the dominant value system. When this language is used by social scientists it functions in the same way. Sociologists' failure to explore the semantic field of their subjects' works against those who have the smallest roles in constructing both popular and scholarly predefinitions. Aging women are good examples of such powerless subjects. . . .

Today the women's movement, even among older women, is organizing and articulating issues and problems that have existed for years. Many of the concerns these women share indicate their rejection of the dominant value system. To decipher such cleavages before they gain widespread and loud expression requires special sensitivity. This sensitivity can be most easily achieved by initially abandoning theoretical assumptions about what should be happening, as well as leaving behind predefined variables, categories, and definitions in favor of an inductive exploration of the symbolic world of the aging woman.

Editor's Conclusion

Who is right, Martin, Kline, or Beeson? Probably, to an extent, all three and equally probably, none of them. Males and females are different, but there are certainly also great differences between individuals within each sex group, differences that all three seem to deemphasize.

We note at least one problem in the data presented by Beeson on the great attachment to work roles by women who retire. One might question whether it is appropriate to compare women who work steadily and full-time with all men of the same status. It would seem on almost *a priori* grounds that most retired men are likely to be married and that most retired women (that is, women who consider their primary role to be that of retired worker, not wife and homemaker) to be never-married, or long-term postmarried. The proper control group for them is not "retired men," but retired men of the same marital status.

Margaret Mead (1949) once hypothesized that some men and women seem to innately fit well into traditional sex roles and others do not. Those whose fit between personality and tradition is good are likely to act as Kline hypothesizes; where the fit is not felicitous as Beeson hypothesizes. In any case, in a society changing its ideas about what is "inherently" male or female as rapidly as ours, by the time we have decided what kinds of people, both male and female, fit well into various roles of today's society, the society will have changed and the problems will also change. All that can happen is that changing one set of circumstances may alleviate one set of problems, but other problems will necessarily arise out of the solution.

Polemics are counterproductive; global hypotheses are equally futile, whether based on "sexist" or "antisexist" stereotypes. It would be more fruitful to inquire what are the characteristics of people (male and female) who adapt easily or with greater difficulty to the new status of retirement. Polemicizing is more fun than that—also easier.

8

What Can We Learn about Aging from Other Places?

So we'll go no more a-roving,
So late into the night
Byron

Editor's Introduction

Societies and cultures are "of a piece" (Benedict, 1934); one aspect
cannot be abstracted out of one society, transplanted into another,
and be expected to perform as it did in the old. Indeed, we cannot
even be sure that cultures are as anthropologists describe them.
Thus, a society described by one observer (Mead, 1935) is startlingly
different than the same data reviewed by other anthropologists
(Winston, 1934, Thurnwald, 1936). It seems that the German rats
and the American rats earlier noted raise their ugly heads whenever
human beings with different world outlooks, philosophies, perhaps
even temperaments, attempt to describe the "objective" reality "out
there."

Attitudes toward and treatment of the aging cannot be taken
out of cultural context (Cowgill and Holmes, 1972). Universally,
long life is valued; few choose to die young, though the age at which
one enters into the status of "aged" varies from one society to the
next. As one ages, one tends to assume more sedentary, advisory,
and supervisory tasks and is normally permitted to lessen involvement in roles involving physical exertion. Children and extended
families undertake responsibility for care of aged kin, even in the
modern industrial society where, the myth has it, such relationships
are passé.

The "problem" of aging has arisen as a direct result of modernization, that is, the twin processes of urbanization and industrialization. In preindustrial societies, life may not always be nasty

127

and brutal, but it is always short, and very few people live to old age. Because these societies, or at least the greater part of their people, are preliterate as well as preindustrial, and technological and social change are glacially slow, the aged have an important function; they are repositories of knowledge, magical rituals, religion, history, and the wisdom of long experience in, at best, a harsh world. In addition, the elders either own or control the use of property. They may not always be loved, but they are revered and respected, because they possess both authority and power.

In our industrial and postindustrial society, the aged are largely redundant. First of all, they are no longer 2–4% of the population, they are well over 10%, up to 13 and 15% in the Scandinavian lands and Austria. Their knowledge and skills soon become obsolete in a rapidly changing society, and who needs the wisdom of just anybody who happens to live long, when one has a library card? The loss of residential stability has weakened the extended family and a money economy has eliminated for all but the aristocracy the power the aged have over others. Those who have worked for large corporations with good pensions and some free professionals whose earnings were high enough to accumulate substantial savings enjoy a golden age as long as they are healthy; for the rest—well, they are the social "problem." This picture is, of course, overdrawn. In times of famine, the old (and the very young) had to be sacrificed in preindustrial society and the modern world retains enough of the old traditions to succor the aged both through public action via social insurances and through the human ties that bind most parents and their adult children. In addition, some older people are wise as well as knowledgeable, having learned something in a lifetime in this world of travail and tears.

This chapter presents attitudes toward social welfare and the aged in Scandinavia and Japan, two very different yet very modern lands. Sweden's modernization process has been more gradual than Japan's, though both are often extolled for their compassion toward the aged.

Editor's Comment: Social Philosophy of Sweden

Many gerontological studies extol the care that the aged receive in the social democracies of Scandinavia and exhort us to act similarly in the United States. However, it is not the aged alone, nor the poor alone, nor any other group, that is singled out for preferential treatment. Care of the aged is merely one aspect of the Scandinavian view of the relationships between the individual, family, state, and people that influence all aspects of social provision in these countries. Our Anglo-American welfare tradition (Axinin and Levin, 1975) grew out of the tradition of the Elizabethan poor laws of 1601, imported to America by both New England dissenter and Southern Anglican establishment types. Thus tradition was one of "residual" welfare services, that is, social services were to be provided only as a last resort, after all family, neighbor, and informal community aid had been exhausted; it was to be the minimal amount necessary to exist, to be given for as short a time as was absolutely necessary and under demeaning circumstances, lest unworthy "sturdy beggars" be tempted to become wards of the state. It was to be locally administered, by the smallest possible unit of government (whose officials presumably knew who were the worthy and unworthy poor), and wherever possible the Poorhouse was the preferred method of succor. In effect, poverty was a crime and punishment for being poor was administered in what was, in effect, a prison. This system lasted in England until the Reforms of 1910–1911 and was ended by those fiery radicals, Lloyd George and Winston Churchill (de Schweinitz, 1943). Only a generation later did Franklin Roosevelt's New Deal begin to make a dent in the Elizabethan tradition in the United States; World War II ended the New Deal and the Viet Nam War ended the Great Society, so America still struggles under the shadow of laws codified in 1601.

By contrast, the Northern European tradition, notably the Scandinavian, has espoused an "institutional" approach to social welfare. Social welfare is available as needed (that is the ideal; in practice, supply does not always meet needs in any society's insatiable demands) for health, welfare, and education to all with no investigation into ability to pay, residence, or other conditions. Services are as freely available as is public education or the library. This simplifies administration enormously. There is no prying into income, other working members of the family, responsibility that can be assumed by unwilling relatives. Nobody is grilled about the need for children's education here and that is how social services are generally administered in Scandinavia (Kammerman and Kahn, 1975). Imagine what a mess it would be if people had to prove their eligibility for public education. To bring birth certificates, pay stubs, utility and rent bills, and so on at regular intervals; to have one's children abruptly taken out of the public school and enrolled in a private school with a rise in income and returned as a work layoff, illness, or other misfortune transfers children back to the stigmatized "poor school." This would make a mockery of education, as it does in public daycare and other services.

These different approaches to social welfare grow out of differing social philosophies. We Americans are rugged individualists, despite the change from the small town craftsman and independent yeoman farmer to the cog in the bureaucratic machine. Social services are given sparingly, grudgingly, a bit nastily lest we tempt the recipient to become a "welfare bum." The Scandinavian philosophy is expressed in the following sections of a paper on Swedish treatment of criminals (Friday, 1976). Nothing has come to our attention that expresses the Scandinavian attitudes toward social welfare as well and succinctly.

Sanctioning in Sweden: An Overview

P. Friday

The places in the world where it is possible for an individual to live a life free from hunger and premature death and where the United Nations Declaration of Human Rights is followed by the governments as something quite self-evident are not many, but Scandinavia, in general, and Sweden, in particular, belong to them. Sweden is often cited as an example of future trends in criminal policy and is often praised (or criticized) for the high standards of the conditions in institutions such as cleanliness, private rooms, the leave system, etc. But they are merely reflections of the general high standard of living in the Swedish society as a whole.

The Swedish penal policy is a reflection of the society as a whole. Both the premises and structure of substantive and procedural laws and of the penal institutions cannot be viewed independently of the values and philosophies of the society itself. . . . Sweden's penal and legal philosophy has developed out of a general social welfare ideology which tends to emphasize the similarities among its citizens rather than the differences.

The fact that Sweden has had a history of peace since the early 19th century and has been ruled by the Social Democrats for more than two generations has promoted social welfare and economic equality. The acceptance of the social welfare policies of the Social Democrats by all political parties is a reaffirmation of the idea that society has a responsibility for the welfare of its members—a tradition more than 200 years old.

Social welfare, Swedish-style, involves more than creating favorable economic conditions. As the late Prime Minister Hansson had suggested, the underlying philosophy behind the welfare system is that the whole country is looked upon as a "folkhemmet," and citizens as members of one family in that home (Marnell, 1972). Of course, this is an ideal which can never be reached, but it has had an important impact on Swedish social thinking and sense of collective responsiblity. The philosophy is not "the survival of the fittest (or richest)" but the "right to survival." The philsophy emphasizes the qualities that people have in common rather than those which make people different. The consequence is the protection of the rights of the weaker members of the society, including those of offenders. A society without slums cannot let their prisoners live under slum conditions; a society which has accepted collective responsibility for the physical and economic welfare of its citizens cannot abuse the rights of even those who transgress against its rules. . . .

Underlying and serving as a basis for relations within Swedish prisons is humaneness and a respect for the individual. Norval Morris' characterization of the system in this regard 10 years ago is still apropos. It is his impression that the Swedish social and political system is pervaded by

> a high level of respect for individual human rights . . . .[Sweden] is . . . a very polite society in which citizens treat citizens and the state treats its citizens with punctilious respect. These attitudes lie deep in Swedish social organization and are in no way abandoned when the citizen becomes a criminal or a prisoner. . . . This humanitarian and egalitarian attitude is indeed the mainspring of the whole correctional system, an explanation of both the low incidence of imprisonment and of many of the conditions and practices within the prison system. . . .
>
> [The average Swedish citizen insists that] the Swedish criminal or prisoner still remains a Swedish citizen meriting respect, continuing properly to enjoy a quite high standard of living and remaining a part of the community. These sentiments are brought to his work by the prison officer who sees a Swedish quality of firm, decent, respectful, and polite treatment between individuals as properly determining his attitude and behavior towards the inmate. It is a great asset, substantially diminishing the alienating prison subculture creating processes that are to be found so often in other countries (Morris, 1966, pp. 48–49)

Editor's Comment

Despite these idyllic descriptions of penology in Sweden, all is not rosy. Though there are only a few thousand people incarcerated there at any one time and most of those are short-termers, such as drunken drivers, there is an irreducible minimum of "hard core" criminals, whom their prison system is incapable of rehabilitating. These constitute about 10% of the prison population (300–400 at a time), who have received indeterminate sentences of up to twelve years, subject to judicial review after the third year and annually thereafter. There are two maximum-security prisons, with all the bars, walls, and locks with which we are familiar, and there are also Swedes who agitate for abolition of the prison system. (Serrill, 1977). Utopias may not be possible in this world, no matter how noble our intentions may be.

Sweden's aged are similarly well cared for. But the generous provision of services solves no problems. The ever-growing number and proportion of the very old swamps the facilities. Despite widespread and well-accepted home-helps (Kammerman and Kahn, 1975), and facilities providing four times as many places in aged homes and six times as many in nursing homes as in Britain, there are long waiting lists and serious shortages of service relative to need (discussion by Middleton in Brocklehurst, 1977).

Contrast with the United States.   The United States is a most reluctant welfare state. We lack the Swedish concept of "folkhemmet" (that is, the country is the home of all its people and every member of the nation has its place in that home). We have argued elsewhere (Wershow, 1979) that the decency of the Scandinavian social democracies lies at least in part in their ethnic homogeneity. They are small countries and lack the American historical experience. Our poor and "dirty workers" were never "of us." They were slaves, indentured servants, uncouth peasants from Ireland, Bohemia, and Italy, Russian Jews and today are likely to be Hispanics, blacks, and Appalachian whites. The post–World War II prosperity has created a similar situation in Northern Europe; their dirty work is now performed by Turks, Yugoslavs, Arabs, Greeks, and other darker people living in poor lands around the Mediterranean sea. And the great enthusiasm for social programs has petered out. Why support so generously these who are not part of the "folk"? In addition, of course, the decline of the work ethic makes the idea of a punitive welfare "stick" attractive in order to discipline a work force that is perceived to be indolent and unamenable to the enticements of the high-wage "carrot."

Editor's Bridging Comment: Policy toward Aging in Japan

Japan is reputed to have retained traditional values toward the aged, despite (or more likely because of) its most rapid modernization. In the next paper Palmore (1975a) presents a view of the Japanese treatment of the aged and what it can teach Americans, followed by comments from reviews of his book on the same subject (Palmore, 1975b), which cast some doubt on his observations.

What Can the USA Learn from Japan about Aging?

E. Palmore

Status and Integration

Aging in Japan is almost a mirror image of aging in the United States. Despite high levels of industrialization and urbanization, the Japanese have maintained a high level of respect for their elders and a high level of integration of their elders in the family, work force, and community. While there is considerable prejudice and discrimination against the aged in America (Palmore, 1969, 1973), old age is recognized by most Japanese as a source of prestige and honor. The most common word for the aged in Japanese, Otoshiyori, literally means "the honorable elders." Respect for the elders is shown in the honorific language used in speaking to or about the elders; rules of etiquette which give precedence to the elders in seating arrangements, serving order, bathing order, and going through doors; bowing to the elders; the national holiday called Respect for Elders Day;

giving seats on crowded public vehicles to the elders; and the authority of the elders over many family and household matters.

The high level of their integration into Japanese society is demonstrated by the following facts. Over 75% of all Japanese aged 65 or more live with their children (Office of the Prime Minister, 1973) in contrast to 25% in the United States (Epstein and Murray, 1967). The majority of Japanese men over 65 continue to be in the labor force (Japan Census Bureau, 1965), compared to 29% of men in the United States over 65 (Palmore, 1964). Most of the Japanese elders who are not actually employed continue to be useful in housekeeping, child-care, shopping, and gardening, often freeing their daughters or daughters-in-law for employment outside the home. The vast majority of Japanese elders also remain active in their communities through Senior Citizens Clubs, religious organizations, and informal neighborhood groups. And, most surprising of all, there appears to have been little decline in these high levels of integration during the past twenty or thirty years (Palmore, 1975b).

This high status and integration of the elders has roots in the "vertical" structure of the society and in the religious principles of filial piety. Japan has often been called a "vertical society" because most relationships tend to be hierarchical rather than horizontal or equalitarian (Nakane, 1972). Age grading is one of the most important dimensions determining who is above or below. The principles of filial piety go back to both Confucian precepts and to ancestor worship, "the real religion of Japan" (Hearn, 1955). The principles of filial piety specify that respect and duty toward parents is one of the most important virtues of all.

Thus, the most general thing we can learn about aging from the Japanese is that high status and integration can be maintained in a modern industrialized society.

Suggestions for the United States and the West

Obviously, many of the practices and attitudes of Japanese toward their elders are not likely to be imported as such. However, many of these practices do suggest ways in which the situation of older Americans in the United States as well as the Western world could be improved.

(1) Respect for the Elders Day is a popular national holiday and apparently succeeds in encouraging respect for the elders and a greater awareness of their problems, as well as actions to reduce these problems. Labor Day and Veterans Day in the United States are similar national holidays which recognize the contributions of labor and veterans as well as encouraging more recognition of their problems. Mother's Day and

Father's Day in the United States are not official government holidays but are widely observed in a variety of ways to recognize the contributions of mothers and fathers. Thus, there seems to be ample precedent for establishing an Older Americans Day in the United States which would be similar in function to Japan's Respect for Elders Day. One difficulty is that while laborers, veterans, mothers, and fathers are generally proud, or at least not ashamed, of their status, many older Americans are ashamed of their status and try to deny their old age. Presumably, if an Older Americans Day could be established, it would help reduce this shame about old age.

(2) The Japanese also use the 61st birthday as an occasion to honor the elders and to express affection for them. In the United States, Americans sometimes use the 21st birthday as an occasion to recognize the new adult. Other rites of passage for the young are christening, confirmation or bar mitzvah, graduation, and marriage ceremonies. There are few such ceremonies for older persons. Sometimes a golden wedding anniversary (after 50 years of marriage) becomes an occasion for recognizing and showing affection for older couples. Sometimes retirement parties are held to recognize an employee's contribution. It might also be useful for the Americans to observe the 65th birthday with special celebrations in order to encourage more respect and affection for our elders.

(3) In an egalitarian society, it is unlikely the West would adopt forms of deference toward older people such as bowing and honorific language. Nevertheless, we do have a weak tradition of "age before beauty" when going through doors and when serving people. This saying, unfortunately, implies that the aged are not beautiful. However, it may be that strengthening and extending the tradition of precedence for older persons would help restore more respect for elders and more self-respect among older persons themselves.

(4) The United States also has a weak tradition of giving seats to elders on crowded public transportation. This could be reinforced, as the Japanese have done, by regulations which give priority to older persons for a certain number of seats in each bus or train. In addition to recognizing special privileges for elders, this would facilitate the ease of travel of older persons, more of whom must rely exclusively on public transportation.

(5) All older Japanese are eligible for a minimum income payment from the government. While this amounts to little more than pocket money at present, the principle of a minimum income guaranteed by the government for older persons is a good one. As of January, 1974, the United States started a program guaranteeing a minimum income to persons over 65 of $140 per month ($210 for a couple). Thus, the principle

of minimum incomes for the aged has only recently been adopted and the next step would be to raise the level of this minimum from its present poverty level to a more adequate income.

(6)   Several cities in Japan have established programs in which elders living alone are visited or called on a daily basis in order to see if they are all right or need anything. Such a program in the United States, which is sporadically conducted instead of being universal, would not only reduce the fears of older persons living alone that they might have some kind of accident or even die before anyone could be reached, but it would also reduce their isolation. . . .

(7)   It is a widespread practice for Japanese of all ages to begin their day with some kind of group exercise. This is carried over into homes for the aged in which the day typically begins with a combination of group exercise and folk dance in rhythm to music. Such morning exercise is widely recognized as an excellent way to preserve physical and mental functioning. When it is done on a group basis, there is the added satisfaction of social support and interaction. Instituting such programs of exercise for older people in the West should improve their physical and mental health (Palmore, 1970; Palmore and Luickart, 1972).

(8)   The Japanese government encourages and subsidizes sports day for the elders. Generally, this takes the form of various track and field events which are not too strenuous for healthy older persons. If the USA government encouraged and subsidized such sports days for older Americans, this too should improve the physical and mental health of those who participate.

(9)   Another program to improve the health of Japanese elders is the free annual health examination, which is followed by more detailed examinations and treatments for those who need it. The present Medicare program in the United States does not cover such routine examinations. It would seem that with only a modest cost to the program, it could be extended to cover an annual examination in order to detect and prevent the development of many serious diseases.

(10)   Starting in 1973, the Japanese government began providing completely free medical care to most Japanese over age 70. Some cities provide free medical care to their residents between the ages of 65 and 70. The present Medicare program in the United States covers only 40% of the medical care cost of older Americans (although other public programs cover another 24%) (Cooper and Piro, 1974). Completely free medical care would remove the high financial barriers that remain between many older people in the USA and adequate medical care. This would not only improve the health of people in the USA and thus improve their life

satisfaction directly, but it would also prevent the depletion of financial resources which so often results from the expenses of serious illness.

(11)   Perhaps the most important single idea the United States could benefit by is the provision of more employment opportunities for older persons. Japanese older persons are not only permitted, but are expected to continue working or doing housework of some kind as long as they are able. There are many ways one could expand job opportunities for older USA people to approach those in Japan. The 1973 White House Conference on Aging recommended the USA earmark a minimum amount of federal manpower funds to improve employment opportunities for older workers; that the USA vigorously enforce and extend the present legislation against discrimination in employment; that the government become the "employer of last resort" for those older workers unable to find other jobs; and that the government establish a computerized national "job bank" and work-related centers to locate and bring together older persons and potential employers on both a full-time and part-time basis (White House Conference on Aging, 1973). During the three years following this conference, none of these recommendations have been carried out. The Japanese believe that voluntary employment of older persons contributes to their physical and mental health, to their satisfaction, to their financial independence, and to the nations's productivity. There is considerable evidence in Japan and in the USA that they are correct in this belief (Palmore, 1972, 1974b).

(12)   Another idea with potentially great benefit is more integration of older persons in the families of their children and grandchildren. It appears unlikely that USA citizens will greatly increase the proportions of older persons living with their children. But it may be feasible and desirable for more older Americans to live near enough to their children and grandchildren to contribute more fully to their household activities. On the one side, this would decrease the isolation and inactivity of many older persons, and on the other side it would reduce the mother's and father's burdens of child care, housekeeping, and household maintenance.

(13)   The Japanese have a nation-wide system of government-supported Elders' Clubs, to which about half the elders belong. These clubs function not only to provide community service, group study, and recreation, but also provide mutual support and self-pride among the elders. The USA has some Senior Citizens' Clubs and some get modest government support. But, compared to Japan, these clubs are few and weak. The National Institute of Senior Aging estimates that less than 5% of Americans over 65 belong to any such club. If the USA follows Japan's example and establishes more, and more active, Senior Citizens' Clubs,

the benefits of greatly expanded community service as well as providing opportunities for group study and recreation, mutual support, and self-pride to the majority of our older citizens would be reaped.

(14)   A related program in Japan is the building of welfare centers for the aged, where various educational, recreational, and consultation services are provided with little or no charge. The centers are subsized by the government and now exist in most large communities. Again, while the USA has a few such centers, they are rare compared to the Japanese. The 1973 White House Conference on Aging recommended:

> In every community and neighborhood, as appropriate, there should be a multipurpose senior center to provide basic social services, as well as link all older persons to appropriate sources of help, including home-delivered services. The basic services, in clearly identifiable sites, i.e., senior centers, action centers, department of social services, etc., financed as an on-going government program, could be the foundation for such additional services as various levels of government and the voluntary sector, including organizations of the aged, would desire and sponsor.

So far, this recommendation has not been officially implemented.

(15)   Perhaps most important in terms of getting these and other recommendations implemented is organized political action and demonstrations by the aged. In Japan, the elders are a recognized political force. This is true not only because they themselves constitute a sizeable proportion of the voters, but because they exert a strong influence over the votes of their family and younger friends. Furthermore, because of the high level of organization and self-pride among the elders, they are able to mount massive demonstrations and other forms of political pressure to get the government to meet their needs better. There are signs in the USA that more of the aged are beginning to realize the necessity for developing more political "clout." They are joining and working though such organizations as the American Association of Retired Persons and the National Council on the Aging in ever-increasing numbers. But massive demonstrations and effective political pressure is still rare. Older people in the USA could learn from their Japanese counterparts more effective ways of organizing and applying political pressure to improve their situation.

(16)   Finally, the most complex and yet fundamental way in which one could learn from the Japanese relates to respect for elders and self-respect among the elders. Respect for Japanese elders is rooted in the basic social structure of their "vertical society" and in their religion of ancestor worship and filial piety. But the very idea of a vertical society and of ancestor worship would seem alien, if not completely repugant to most

USA citizens. Yet it appears that respect for the aged is the key element which can maintain the status and integration of the aged in modern industrial societies. Therefore, in order to improve the status and integration of older Americans, it is necessary to improve respect for the aged somehow. Instead of the vertical society, perhaps one could use egalitarian ideology that all persons are entitled to respect because they are humans, regardless of race, sex, or age. Instead of ancestor worship, perhaps one could use the Judaic-Christian commandment, "Honor thy father and mother," to increase respect for the aged. Perhaps the beliefs that "experience is the best teacher" and that knowledge can come from books but only years of experience can provide wisdom can be revived. Whatever the method or ideological base, it seems probable that respect for older Americans must be substantially increased before their status and integration will be substantially increased.

The commentary above is not intended to propose a culture which assumes the aged are superior simply because they are old (as was true in old Japan). Nor is this intended to be an argument for a gerontocracy in which the aged have most of the power and rewards of the society (as in ancient Japan). It is intended, instead to suggest that stereotypes and prejudices in the USA and other Western countries should be overcome to provide the elderly equal respect with all other humans; and, therefore, in the USA discrimination against the aged in employment, in our families, and in our communities should be stopped so that they can regain an equal share of power and rewards.

Those who agree with these ideals may be able to learn something from the land of The Honorable Elders.

On the Other Hand—Some Contrary Views of Aging in Japan

From a review of The Honorable Elders
by T. Chadwick (1976)

But Palmore falls short of substantiating his first theory, ignoring many facts, and relying on a romanticized wish that there really is an exception to the theory that modernization and decline in the status of the elderly correspond strongly. Or if there is an exception, Japan is not it. . . . Palmore mentions instances over and over again that point to the steady decline in the status of Japanese elderly. Furthermore, Japanese gerontological and social welfare literature stresses that the situation of the elderly is worsening, that the gap between the strong legislatively-mandated Preamble of the Welfare for the Aged Law and actual practice is just as wide in Japan as in the USA. While Palmore bases much of his argument on overt aspects of respect toward the elderly, aspects which are embedded in a slowly-changing language and present in 2000 years of religious thought and activity, the Tokyo Metropolitan Government states that in recent years families have become less considerate of the elderly and that 48.9% of Tokyo aged living with their families worry about their health and survival because their families do not take good care of them (Ministry of Health and Welfare, 1974). . . . Palmore cites the statistic that three-fourths of Japanese elders 65+ live with their children, and says that he has seen no data on the economic necessity of the generations living together. Yet Broberg, Melching, and Maeda (1975) says the only reason the dislocation of the elderly in favor of nuclear family-living by the young is not happening faster is the underdeveloped funding of social insurance and the severe housing shortage. Palmore presents *evidence* through his Equality Index to show that Japanese elderly are more integrated into the work force than the elderly of other industrialized nations, ignoring the need for similarity in comparisons, for in most other industrialized nations the elderly are kept out of employment because there aren't the type of jobs which keep the Japanese elderly employed such as street peddling, work in small shops, and field work. Those Japanese who work after the retirement age of 55 do so at vastly reduced pay scales, forfeiting all seniority, while they are not eligible for retirement benefits until the age of 65.

Since Palmore, himself, cites many cases indicating the decline in status of the elderly, he seems to make his arguments through the romanticism of rose-colored glasses. The most that can be said is that the decline in the status of the elderly in Japan has been occurring at a slower rate than the modernization and aging theory would indicate. There are also other factors besides culture that may be affecting the decline in the status of the elderly. When the Japanese began to industrialize at the beginning of the century they decided to learn about the best and worst consequences of industrialization from the experiences of other countries. One of those consequences was the decline in the status of the aged. As a result, Japan began very early to plan ways to slow, or prevent, the decline in the status of Japanese elderly. As the Japanese are the first to admit, they have not succeeded in preventing the trend, but they have laid a very extensive, if underfunded, framework which has as its goal the maintenance of respect and standard of living for the elderly.

From a review of The Honorable Elders
by M. Riley (1976)

The Honorable Elders poses important questions. Is the traditional culture in Japan a stronger force than the Japanese economy in determining the position of the elderly, as Palmore would have us believe? Or, we might ask, is this merely an instance of cultural lag, in a nation caught midway in a rapid process of industrialization that will predictably undermine both tradition and the status of the aged? Palmore offers some new data, but they provide mixed evidence. Although he asserts that "the status of Japanese elders has suffered little decline," many of his statements seem to support the alternative hypothesis of transitional decline. Some statements indeed imply this decline: "much of this tradition is being . . . rejected by the younger generation"; "support patterns show a trend away from family support"; "the proportion of Japanese over 60 living with their children [has] declined." Other statements indicate that the old are not yet primarily involved in the industrial sector: "the older people have tended to stay on the farms and in the fishing villages. . . . This is [related to] their high rate of continued employment"; a table shows that old people are more likely to live with children in rural areas than in large cities. Some of Palmore's evidence, like that reported by Ruth Benedict for the 1940s, seems irrelevant for the current stage in the transition. And some, like the appropriation by the young of the elderly's "silver seats" on the railroad, seems to negate his argument entirely. Most disconcerting is the disregard of the age structure of the population which, because of rapid demographic change, is likely to contain more of the "young old"—the more competent—than of the "old old". . . .

There are other traces of perfunctory scholarship. "Conclusions" are asserted even when evidence is slim. Thus "the Japanese elders appear to be as healthy or healthier than older Americans"—yet the chapter on health notes only that life expectancy is similar, while discounting Japan's comparatively higher rates of suicide and of the housebound. There are misreadings of the American data used as a foil for the Japanese. Thus "older Japanese have less leisure time than older Americans"—yet the American sample is both older and less economically active than the Japanese sample.

From a review of The Honorable Elders
by A. McCord (1976)

[I]f the elderly live such a happy life why does the suicide rate in Japan spurt upwards at age 55? In America, suicide for males also increases at this age but it *declines* for American females. In Japan, rates of suicide more than quadruple for both males and females after age 55. If the "honorable elders" in Japan are so extraordinarily respected and active, why do they take their lives more often in old age than similar people in other industrialized nations? It may well be that an ancient Japanese stereotype holds true: the old are tolerated and paid outward respect, yet they (particularly mothers-in-law who move in with their children) are actually resented.

Editor's Comment

Plath (1972) emphasizes the ambiguity and ambivalence toward the aged of Japanese society. While the aged are formally honored, they are also, as the reviews cited shows, probably not much less neglected than in the USA, and ageism does exist in Japan. The high suicide rate among the aged is partly explained by an aspect of the Japanese mores, which admires suicide as the supreme moral act of self-sacrifice for the benefit of the larger group. Even honorable elders' suicides are deemed praiseworthy when their continued existence becomes destructive to self and society. Suicide may be encouraged by the feelings (which coexist with the obligation of filial support) that being old is a "Hateful Age"; the negative features are reinforced by low income due to forced retirement at an early age, with the concomitant loss of company-provided benefits: low cost housing and recreational facilities and clubs, which provide a home away from the small, overcrowded Japanese urban apartment. Japan is currently moving rapidly from some preindustrial forms to which the society remained committed as long as possible. The current cohort of aged, as Plath puts it, "have been turned loose into new lifespan territory. It has equipped them only with medieval maps, full of freaks and monsters and imaginary harbors. The aged are among the true pioneers of our time, and pioneer life is notoriously brutal" (p. 150).

Editor's Conclusion

Certainly not all of Palmore's list of suggestions are translatable to the American scene. Special days and birthdays cannot be lifted out of context. In America, vigorous attempts to celebrate Senior Citizens Week has resulted in public officials signing proclamations and some publicity, which may be somewhat more meaningful than National Pickle Week. But even Mother's Day (and who in America is holier than Mom?) has benefited the greeting card and chocolate bon-bon producers much more than mothers. Some of Palmore's examples receive greater praise than their Japanese context warrants; for example, "several cities in Japan" have what we call "reassurance service" to elderly. But the United States is scolded because our services are "sporadically conducted instead of being universal."

Anderson (1976) points out, in an excellent discussion, that we are unlikely to adequately provide for the neediest group of aged, that is, the 10–15% who are severely disabled (two-thirds of whom are not in institutions) and who require a great deal of expensive care. This greatly debilitated group is least likely to become politically active, nor are their children or other concerned caretakers likely to be able to take the time from their burdensome duties to conduct political activity. As Binstock (1978) in the paper to be cited shows, we will probably continue to piddle huge sums away "here and there" with no idea of providing more adequately for services ranked in any reasonable order of priority.

Besides, who engages in "massive demonstrations" in the United States? Japanese may, for better or worse, carry out bloody riots to prevent building the new Tokyo airport, nuclear power plants, etc. In the United States, we can count massive political activities of recent years on two fingers: Dr. Martin Luther King, Jr.'s civil rights march on Washington and the public outrage at Nixon's secret raids on Cambodia. We are neither Japanese nor Europeans, and our traditions are different.

Using this example from Japan, we can see that any one person's view of reality may not necessarily be the whole picture. Palmore is probably partly correct in his assessment of Japanese society. It probably has retained many preindustrial features. But the evidence, even as he presents it, is not clear-cut. How much might his perceptions have been influenced by nostalgia, by his memories of "coming home" to the country where he grew up in a missionary family? We don't know and he doesn't know, as who among us can accurately assess his own motivation.

Recommended Readings

Cowgill, D. and Holmes, L., eds. *Aging and Modernization*. New York: Appleton-Century-Crofts, 1972.

Kammerman, S. and Kahn, A. *Not for the Poor Alone: European Social Services*. Philadelphia: Temple University Press, 1975.

Simic, A. "Aging in the U.S. and Yugoslavia: Contrasting Models of Intergenerational Relationships." *Anthropological Quarterly* 50 (1977): 53–64.

Part Five
Policy and Service Issues

9

Issues of Public Policy: How Do We Best Serve the Elderly?

Nothing is easier than spending public money. It does not appear to belong to anybody. The temptation is overwhelming to bestow it on somebody.

Calvin Coolidge, quoted in Laurence J. Peter, *Peter's Principles: Ideas for Our Time*

Editor's Introduction

The quotation from Calvin Coolidge is not meant to signal our application for membership in the John Birch Society, but to point up the fundamental question: What do you do when you don't have enough to do everything everybody wants done, even to do everything that a consensus of our citizenry would agree needs to be done desperately? This and another issue are the two major issues in public policy discussions, the other being: How can any bureaucratic organization become as efficient, as cost-conscious, as intimately linked to satisfied customers, while maintaining economies of large scale organization, as was the corner grocery store my father ran? The question applies as much to private as to public bureaucracies. It's nobody's money, and nobody either visibly suffers or gains when employees loaf, are insolent to the public, or even steal. The ques-

147

tion is equally valid in all political and economic systems; only true believers of one stripe or another will attempt to deny it. Unfortunately the first question is usually ignored and the second goes unasked. Thus, in the entire issue of *The Gerontologist* devoted to "Aging in the Year 2000" (Neugarten, 1975), not one paragraph is devoted to the prospect that we may not be able to always provide more and more and more of better and better. Few have considered the problems raised by Wershow (1973b, 1979), Rosow (1975), and Club of Rome (1972) that treat the impending problems and the dangers that will confront people in the twenty-first century if present trends go unchecked.

Following a short excerpt from Rosow, we move on to a discussion of priority-setting in a British context by Arie (1977) and thence to a discussion of federal spending and planning for the aged. Planning is, unfortunately, no more than a minor aspect of the political process of governmental activity at any level. I once asked an official of the Administration of Aging if any planning was being done for those who will be aged in the year 2000. After all, they have all been born already and we know not only how many they will be, but how much education they will have had, their occupational level, and other information. His answer was, "Don't be naive. This is an election year and nobody in Washington is planning beyond November." The effects of the American way of running a country is shown in a paper by Binstock (1978). After that macrolevel approach, a paper is presented (Tobin and Thompson, 1975) that questions, on the level of the small service agency, whether the hue and cry about accountability has not led to an overemphasis on "countability." The problem of reaching the hard-to-reach, whose service needs are greatest, is lost in the emphasis on cost-benefit ratios, that is, one gets funded and refunded by serving many rather than the neediest.

A discussion questioning our "liberal" emphasis on progressive tax structures (Wilensky, 1978) ends the chapter on a matter of great importance to gerontology. Most services to older people are likely to be public, tax-supported services. It behooves us to think about ways of raising funds that are best accepted by the taxpayers, and progressive taxes may not be the answer.

The Aged in Post-Affluent Society

I. Rosow

These conditions [characteristic of post-industrial society] are endemic to the proliferation of modern industrialism, pressures to maximum economic growth, and the unprecedented demographic survival rates. They are fostered by almost insatiable popular aspirations for ever-higher living standards, invariably accompanied by prodigal consumerism, and other massive wastes. The consequences are to be seen in the objective problems of dwindling natural resources, rising energy requirements, and severe pollution, all intensified by tremendous population pressures. In terms of an economic model, this is analogous to a vast increase in the demand for values and goods in the face of a drastic reduction in their supply.

In other words, during this critical period, we are faced with the prospect of a raging Malthusian-Orwellian world, of rising scarcities and shortages of essentials that may literally wipe out people in unprecedented and unimaginable numbers. The economic and social strains that could result would drastically alter the conditions of man's life and many aspects of social organization. . . .(p. 8)

How might the aged fare in such circumstances? The answer, regrettably, is: not very well. First, as we have indicated, there should be a disproportionate attrition among the elderly during the transitional decades. Life expectancy would decline, and fewer and fewer people should reach old age, especially if there were any serious breakdown in medical services and the drug industry, not to mention the other necessities of life. So the recent demographic trends that have increased the number and proportion of the elderly should be arrested and then reversed. (p. 13)

Editor's Bridging Comment: Priority-Setting

In light of these problems, the questions of priorities in programs for the aged—both the priority to be given to resources devoted to the aged in competition with other interest groups and for various services to the aged—become pressing even now.

The insufficiency of medical care is a good heuristic device to clarify in its starkest reality the problem of priorities, which, on the level of the individual provider and consumer, becomes a problem of rationing scarce resources. We engage in rationing all the time—whenever one person on an agency waiting list receives service and another does not, whenever the budgeting process designates a sum of money for one budgeted item rather than another. However, the problem becomes more starkly visible when life and death matters are at stake. Let Arie (1977) point out the problem from the vantage point of the British National Health Service.

Brain Failure in Old Age:
Thoughts on Rationing and Responsibility

T. H. Arie

I want to speak about two aspects of life in the National Health Service which I will sum up by the not very beautiful but alliterative catchwords, 'Rationing' and 'Responsibility'. In these few minutes one can try only to raise a few issues, rather than to settle any of them.

Rationing, 'Macro' and 'Micro'

The 'rationing' of medical care is on many people's lips these days. . . . Rationing, with its suggestion of the rational, is attractive and brings back memories of wartime, when many people were actually better provided for than before, and others were healthier for eating less.

But do we have a rationed service, or merely a shortage service? So far rationing of medical resources has begun to be attempted only at what one could call the 'macro' level—that is at national, regional, and perhaps area level, though very little yet at the level of the last of these. Contrasted with this 'macro' rationing is rationing at the 'micro' level, which is where clinicians spend their working days. The meaning of 'rationing' in the context of the day-to-day disbursal of resources to individuals is something very different from large-scale decisions about priorities. It is a weary fact that though many may accept that in *general* there is not enough to go round, yet each individual is confident that the demands of any *particular* case in which he has an interest can somehow be met.

Clinicians (and by this I mean not only doctors but all those in the health professions who deal one-to-one with members of the public) are caught between the shearing force of manifest shortage on the one hand, and on the other hand the confident assumption on the part of users of the service that any particular demand must be met on its apparent merits. And by 'users of the service' I mean not only patients, but also colleagues within the service when they are making demands on each other.

In our field of old-age medicine, and in particular of dementia, it is exceedingly unlikely that every demand could ever be met on its merits; and the present state of the economy makes it quite certain that there can be no reason at all to expect that available resources should even approximately match the extent of present demand on them. To believe otherwise is to subscribe to what I call the 'Desiderative Fallacy', instances of which abound in health and social services: one version of this holds that because something needs treatment, therefore there must somewhere be a treatment for it; the supposition that because a situation arises which appears to need certain resources, therefore those resources must somewhere be available, is another instance of the same fallacy. . . .

Doctors are reared to believe that the only consideration in their work should be to do 'what is best for the patient'. This is no ignoble ideal, but unfortunately no-one has prepared us for the discovery that except very occasionally, or in societies where medical care is available only to those who can pay its market cost, it is simply not possible to make a decision about one patient without at the same time implicitly making decisions about other patients. At the 'macro' level to which I have referred, this process is commonly called 'deciding priorities.' But it operates just as surely at the 'micro' level, the level of the individual clinical transaction, for any resources made available to an individual are thereby no longer available to other individuals who either need them, or may shortly do so. A decision to make available a bed or a place in a day hospital means that the bed or that place is no longer there for others; a decision to offer psychotherapy or surgery means that that amount of psychotherapist's or surgeon's time has been withdrawn from the available pool of local manpower.

Similarly a decision to relieve one family's burden by admitting a demented old person to hospital may mean that one is thereby intolerably adding to the burden of the nurses (and other patients) on a short-staffed, and these days often almost unstaffable, long-stay ward. It is fashionable to make a contrast between clinical medicine and community medicine, but there is a sense in which it is impossible equitably to practice the former without at the same time practicing the latter. Or as Lawrence Weed has put it, not to consider the needs of *all* the people, means that most of the people will get a poorer deal.

Doctors have to operate this 'rationing' from a position of double disadvantage; first, their training has ill-prepared them for doing so, or even for recognizing that they *are* doing so; and second unlike wartime rationing, the principles of the rationing which individual doctors have to apply are nowhere publicly stated or officially underwritten. Thus decisions by clinicians are naturally open to question and challenge, and are in fact constantly challenged. And since these challenges are often based on very strong claims, or have loud voices behind them, they are quite likely to be upheld and the decision reversed, if only for the sake of peace. Rarely, if ever, is a local declaration made of what is and what is not available, to which the 'rationer' can appeal. Yet one effect of achieving peace by conceding a resource because of the strength of pressure, rather than on its merits in relation to what is available, is that the real extent of the actual shortage is hidden.

However politically sensitive it might be, the conclusion surely is that *it has now become urgently necessary that in each health district decisions be reached, and openly promulgated, as to what the public can and what it cannot expect from its local health services.* This would not be a static announcement, but would constantly be open to review in the light of changing resources, changing demand, and changing views of priorities. . . . Public pressure and challenge should continue even after agreement has been reached—but it would then be directed against a declared and known consensus, rather than at the judgments of individuals. An added bonus from a public statement of deficiencies would be that they would be there for all to see rather than swept under the carpet—and in that way there would be more chance that they might be remedied, either by local redistribution, or by their manifest nature being a more powerful attractor of resources from without. And at the same time the 'spivs' [British World War II slang for swindlers and black marketeers] who get (or provide) more than is fair would be more readily exposed. (pp. 104–106)

Editor's Bridging Comment:
Are We Serving the Aged Well?

How well do our many programs serve the aged? The American pattern, as Binstock (1978) points out in the following paper, is to provide many programs that are largely symbolic gestures, meant to show that the legislative and executive branches do something, yet that spread very little money too thinly, ignore the most pressing problems, and make no attempt to meet the most pressing needs. In another paper, Binstock (1972) names chapter and verse (and organizations) and details the political processes involved. Indeed, looking at the American system of diffusion of power and control, as well as the chronic shortage of funds and the increasing pressures on necessarily limited and diminishing resources referred to earlier, what other choices exist than to dodge the major problems and to meet some needs with feeble, symbolic gestures and gobs of publicity?

Federal Policy toward the Aged:
Its Inadequacies and its Politics

R. Binstock

The remarkably large proportion of federal spending that is devoted to programs for the elderly is becoming well known. . . . [A]bout one-fourth of the budget for fiscal year 1978 was spent on older persons. Given demographic projections that show continuing increases in the number and proportion of Americans who are 65-years-old and over, Califano and others have emphasized that spending to maintain the current federal mosaic of benefits for the aging could reach more than 40% of total federal expenditures relatively early in the next century.

What has not been emphasized sufficiently, however, is the extent to which the current expenditure of $112 billion on programs for the aging represents an indictment of the American style of domestic public policy. One might expect that if the federal government allocates one-quarter of its budget to a particular target population of 23 million citizens, then that population's economic, health, and social problems would be substantially alleviated. Yet, that is not the case. While significant help is provided to many older persons through federal programs, even more significant problems remain—problems that Congress and the Executive Branch have officially committed us to solving.

How could it be that we are spending so much money on the problems of aging and having only limited success? Is it because we are committed to doing too many things for the aged? If our commitments are overextended to this specific constituency, how generally over-committed are we to solving the problems of the myriad constituencies that have beseiged

Washington and won some form of programmatic acknowledgement that their problems should be solved?

More fundamentally, what style of politics has led us into a situation in which we get such limited results with so many dollars expended on public policies that are expected to alleviate social problems? Is that style likely to change in the foreseeable future? The case of the aging may elicit some useful perspectives on these matters. But before addressing such issues, let us consider the ways in which "the high cost of aging" to the federal treasury is and is not helping older persons.

The Unresolved Problems

Our current agenda of public programs toward the aging is truly incredible for it includes virtually every aspect of human existence. Congress has enacted programs that imply responsibilities to the aging for: adequate income maintenance; health care; nutritional, supportive and leisure services; housing; transportation; protection against crime; legal services; home repair; tax rebates; help in getting jobs; protection against discrimination in employment; and a variety of other matters. In a recent survey of policies affecting aging, the U.S. House of Representatives Select Committee on Aging identified 134 federal "programs benefitting the elderly" under the jurisdiction of 49 congressional committees and subcommittees. If we contemplate the additional universe of major and minor programs generated by the state and local governments in the United States as well as big institutions in the private sector, any desire we may have to undertake a thorough inventory of relevant policies and programs readily disappears.

The sheer number of programs related to aging, or to any other phenomenon in American society is in itself instructive. It readily indicates that issues and problems are easily placed on the agenda as legitimate concerns of government. One seems to need only to state an issue to legitimize it as a public responsibility. On the other hand, it should be equally clear that the mere presence of an issue on the agenda of legitimated public responsibilities in no way can be taken as a sign that the issue will be resolved.

Income security. The federal government has had the most impact in alleviating the problems of aging through efforts to provide income security. . . . [T]he average income situation of older persons has been improved markedly through the impact of social security (OASI), supplemental security income (SSI), and the civil service, military, and railroad retirement programs, combined with pension plans of state and local governments and those in the private sector. Primarily because of dramatic increases in OASI benefits and expenditures during the past decade (from about $25 billion in 1969 to about $90 billion in 1979) the proportion of older persons with incomes below the poverty line has dropped from one in four to one in seven. However, since the poverty line is based on a temporary emergency diet, this leaves some 3.3 million older persons in dire financial circumstances.

The job that still needs to be done to provide a decent measure of income security to the aging can be better understood if we place the poverty line within the context of the slightly higher "near poor line." This measure consists of a series of budgetary indexes based on a permanent "economy" diet. If we use this near poor line, we find that 25% of the aging, or about 5.5 million persons, lack sufficient income to support a minimum adequate permanent diet. In short, the aggregate income condition of the aged has been greatly improved by federal income security programs, but a very large segment within that population remains in severe financial distress.

Health. Receiving less attention than income security in the past few years, and probably far more difficult to deal with in the long run, are issues concerning the improvement of older persons' health. Herman Brotman reported earlier in this *National Journal* series that "older people are subject to more disability, see physicians 50 per cent more often and have about twice as many hospital stays that last almost twice as long as is true for younger persons." But federal expenditures for health care have done little to alleviate the health problems of the aging.

The medicare and medicaid programs enacted in 1965 have helped to defray the costs of seeing doctors, staying in hospitals, and obtaining several additional specific health services and goods. But these programs have not had an impact on the health status of older persons, whether aggregated for all persons 65 and older or disaggregated for different age groups within that population.

The probability of any person being institutionalized at some time in their life after their 65th birthday is 25%, or one in four. And we are much too familiar with the uneven, often scandalous, nature of institutional care, as well as the feckless pattern through which our national and state governments deal with abuses in nursing homes and other long-term care institutions. We have seen often enough the cycle through which media exposure of nursing home conditions engenders a sense of public outrage, a commission is appointed to investigate conditions and to recommend legislation to deal with them and reasonable strong regulatory standards are enacted. Nonetheless, the nursing home industry remains remarkably immune to regulation by neutralizing or capturing the machinery of regulatory implementation.

The highly-touted "alternatives to institutional care"—home health care and homemaker services—are still touted, but not implemented on a substantial scale. One major reason they have not been fully developed is because neither medicare nor medicaid provide for the elements of home service that do not involve a skilled nursing component. Consequently, a great many of the theoretically viable alternatives to institutional care remain financially impracticable. . . .

Social services and facilities. With all the attention that is being directed to the costs of income security and health care programs, other federal programs among the 134 benefitting the aging have hardly been noticed, probably because their budgets are comparatively negligible. Nonetheless, the problems that such programs are supposed to be alleviating are of considerable importance to many older persons and their families.

Perhaps the most useful example is provided by the Older Americans Act of 1965, a legislative omnibus administered by HEW's Administration on Aging (AoA), and costing about $500 million in fiscal year 1978. The range of programs initiated and supported through this act, which was reauthorized and expanded just a few weeks ago, has set forth an extensive agenda of American society's responsibilities toward its older citizens. Through more than a dozen years of legislation and implementation, the Older Americans Act has brought to the fore as legitimate public concerns the need for: home care services, transportation, nutrition, leisure programs, protection against crime, legal services, home repair, regulatory ombudsmen, research and career training in aging, and a variety of other supportive services.

In order to implement programs aimed at these concerns, AoA has elaborated a so-called "national network on aging" anchored by 600 area agencies on aging. The network also includes 1,000 senior centers, 9,000 nutrition program sites where congregate meals are served, and hundreds of public and voluntary service and planning organizations, as well as research and education programs, devoted to concerns of older persons. Without sustenance from the Older Americans Act, most of these operations would not exist or would be devoting their attention and efforts to other matters than aging.

There is no doubt that the programs of the Older Americans Act directly help many older persons through the provisions of a variety of health and social services, free meals, and opportunities to make useful contributions to community life. And there is little question that AoA's nationwide bureaucratic network generates ongoing support for the act and its programs. Almost every congressional district is served by an area agency and has within it some older persons who are benefitting from specific services provided through AoA's programs.

Unfortunately, these positive features of the Older Americans Act go hand-in-hand with a series of weaknesses.

First, the extensive range of programmatic responsibilities has been elaborated without much sense of priority. Consequently, the small amount of available funds is distributed relatively thinly among many objectives and is far from sufficient to make a substantial impact on any given problem.

A second and related weakness is that the programmatic agenda and bureaucratic network have been developed with sufficient fanfare to create a cruel illusion that a variety of problems can eventually be solved through funding and implementation under the Older Americans Act. We can appreciate the extent to which this is an illusion if we consider that no one problem of the many toward which the act's programs are directed could be solved through the present pattern even if funding were drastically increased. For example, according to testimony by a recent director of New York City's Office on Aging, the act's Title VII nutrition program is meeting about 1% of the national need. Are we looking toward an appropriation of over $20 billion that would be required to fund an adequate number of nutrition programs throughout the country? And tens of billions for each of the other programmatic needs?

A third weakness is that the bureaucratic components of the network—the public and voluntary service agencies and the universities and colleges—have quite understandably become preoccupied with sustaining and expanding the different, thinly-funded program elements with which they are directly involved. Each program element has a corresponding set of bureaucratic or educational mechanisms, and each of these sets has developed its own professional organization or association. As a consequence, one finds a great deal of attention given to the apportionment of Older Americans Act funds earmarked for each of the bureaucratic domains in the network, but little, if any, attention to how a given problem confronting older persons is to be solved. . . .

What Style of Politics Gets Us into this Situation?

. . . If this is our record in social policy toward the aging, what is the record in other areas of social policy in which we spend far less? We know the answer too well; our policies of social intervention are frustratingly ineffective. The War on Poverty was not won, but abandoned. The Model Cities program did not produce model cities.

Why is it that American social policies are continually disappointing, with all the dollars we expend through them? There are many factors that can explain our ineffective approaches to social intervention, far too many to begin to consider within the scope of this discussion.

The central point to consider is the obvious one—that most of our public policies are not designed as interventions to solve social problems. Rather, they are enacted and implemented by public officials in a fashion likely to solve the problems of public officials.

To be sure, in the context of a dramatic crisis such as the Great Depression, it is possible for the needs of politicians to be subordinated to the needs of the collectivity. The legislation enacted during the New Deal, especially the Social Security Act of 1935, may provide the best illustration of this phenomenon. However, if one compares OASI and its contributory "insurance" rubric with more radical schemes of the era such as the Townsend Plan, even the original social security program does not seem sharply focused on the solution of income security problems.

Overload of demands. Except in the context of dramatic crises, when personal disaster can strike virtually all strata of society, our public policies are relatively symbolic responses to demands which are made upon the political system. As such, these responses—like the 134 federal programs benefitting the aging—are politically functional for our public officials in that they set a record of concern for the demands that have been made, and thereby cool off the demands. Through this style an overwhelming array of programs is proliferated, but few, if any, problems are solved. . . .

A circuit-breaker formula. Particularly in the area of social services, Congress has developed a "circuit-breaker" formula for coping with this overload of demands, a formula through which it enacts legislation but avoids specific substantive issues of policy implementation. The central ingredient of this circuit-breaker formula, of which the Older Americans Act is a clear example, is a distribution of funds to state and local entities, with only the most general rules about what should be done with the distributed resources. Sometimes the funds are to be distributed to existing entities, but often, the legislation calls for the designation and creation of new entities (such as area agencies on aging) that can be identified through direct symbolism with the issue to which the legislation is responding. The substantive responsibilities of these implementing activities are usually described in the most general of terms: develop services and comprehensive plans; coordinate; undertake advocacy. A flexible, competitive process is established for distributing minor amounts of funds to organizations that are directly engaged in operating programs, and the networks of new entities are urged to compete with each other for additional federal government funds.

The ingredients of this circuit-breaker formula comprise a recipe for political triumph, though not one for effective social intervention. Through the adoption of legislation based on this recipe, national politicians can maintain and reinforce their legitimacy as public leaders. The cadres of state and local entities that receive federal funds, as well as their associated participating constituencies and interest groups, are grateful supporters of the policy although they inevitably regard as inadequate the amount of funds made available to them. Constituencies and interests that are unable to gain access to the resources distributed by such policies decry them, but they tend to be accommodated through inclusion in subsequent amendments.

While legislation is vague about the social outcomes to be achieved through policy, it is relatively specific about the allocation of funds to newly-designated or newly-created implementation entities and their need, in turn, to expend effort to distribute money for developing programs. Consequently, "successful results" can ensue relatively quickly and in tangible form. Virtually all that is required is to report on the number of entities that have been established, and the number of dollars that have been widely distributed among constituencies throughout the nation.

This pattern of political behavior provides an excellent means of responding symbolically to a variety of politicized issues, of setting a record that Congress has done something and cares about the needs of the constituency. But nowhere in this pattern can be found a substantive and financial focus on service priorities that could be taken as even a *prima facie* case that such policies could meet the true need for services.

Income distribution politics. Turning from service policies to look at income transfer programs like OASI [Social Security], we find that the pattern of political action is somewhat different though still not focused sharply on solving older persons' problems of income security. . . . [I]nitiatives and support for social security amendments have been focused on raising benefits and broadening coverage, not on eliminating the severe financial distress which is still experienced by millions of elderly persons.

Our politicians have preferred what they perceive to be a safe course by maintaining a benefit distribution pattern that is reasonably in harmony with the "social insurance" mythology which helped to generate and sustain the political acceptability of the program. In so doing they have created a situation in which almost all older persons are covered by OASI, but with very uneven consequences. Several million older persons with two or more pensions have very comfortable retirement incomes; 5.5

million are in dire financial straits, and the remainder are moderately well-off.

In generating this peculiar distribution of retirement income in the name of providing *income security*, the Congress and presidents have brought us to a situation in which opinion leaders and decision makers are alarmed about the high costs of financing income transfer programs for the aging. Yet, most proposals for reforming OASI have largely focused on methods of restructuring the manner in which the present benefit system is financed, and not on ways of helping the fourth of the older population that is in severe financial distress. Also overshadowed or lost in the current furor over the "graying of the budget" through increased costs of income transfer programs are the challenges that must be faced if we are to keep our commitments to meet the health care and social service implications of an aging population.

What Can Be Done?

Secretary Califano (of the Department of Health, Education, and Welfare) has suggested that we find solutions to the unresolved problems of aging, without substantially increasing the current projected budgetary costs. This is a fitting, statesmanlike challenge for the head of HEW to present. How can it be answered?

Increase efficiency?   Is the limited success of our policies on aging due to programmatic inefficiency? Would we be able to get better results with the same amount of resources if our policies were designed in a more comprehensive, coordinated fashion?

If we were simply looking at health care and social problems, we might be tempted to answer "yes," placing the blame on a patchwork "non-system" for delivering services. But we would be foolish to succumb to this temptation, for the components of the "delivery system" we have in this country include 80,000 distinct governments, thousands of hospitals, nursing homes, and health and social service agencies in both the private and public sector. There is plenty of room for increased efficiency in service delivery, but it is unlikely to be achieved through a national design. It truly boggles the mind to contemplate that some dedicated public servants in the federal government may be trying to design a comprehensive, coordinated delivery system comprised of our incredibly crowded terrain of governments and agencies, let alone trying to implement one from Washington.

If we look at OASI, it is difficult to charge the program with inefficiency. Despite an occasional mistake in the computerized system for issuing checks, the Social Security Administration generally delivers the appropriate amount of benefits to the proper recipients as defined by OASI legislative provisions. . . .[I]t is, after all, OASI which accounts for about 80 per cent of the federal expenditures on the aging. . . .

Await the impact of "senior power"?   Many advocates for the severely disadvantaged aging, recognizing the limited effectiveness of our current policies, have comforted themselves with the notion that "senior power" will sharply increase federal expenditures and administrative efforts to improve the income security, health, and social problems of older persons. Looking to the increases in the numbers and proportion of older voters, they cling to images of the aging as a powerful or soon-to-be powerful voting bloc and organized interest. . . .

Both those who cherish the image of senior power and those who fear it have been misled. Although older persons do cast 15% or more of the vote in national elections, they do not all vote the same. The population of older persons is politically heterogeneous, just as it is economically and socially heterogeneous.

Even if we accept the problematic assumption that voters are swayed by issues favoring their self interest, most older voters do not primarily identify themselves, and hence their self interest, in terms of aging. When a person reaches 65 or enters retirement status, he or she does not suddenly lose all prior self identities—sex, race, education, peer group and community ties—and the self-interests that can be derived from them. . . .

Analyses of age as a variable in political attitudes and voting patterns have consistently shown that the differences within age groups are greater than the differences between age groups. No sound evidence has been assembled showing an instance in which an "old age interest" or an "old age candidate" can be presumed to have shifted older persons' votes as a cohesive force.

Although the commonly purveyed images of the aging as a political force are inaccurate, the images, in themselves, provide resources for some limited forms of power. The image of an aged voting bloc leads many politicians to support propositions that seem favorable to older persons, and to attend sizable meetings that involve older persons and their presumed interests. They do not wish to be listed among "the missing," when the rolls of "supporters of the aging" are compiled. On the other hand, the image of the aging as a voting bloc is not sufficiently powerful to evoke more than moderate, incremental and symbolic support.

The relatively few politicians who make a heavy investment (even a symbolic one) in support for the aging, relative to their support for other constituencies, learn regretfully about the inaccurate image of the aging voting bloc. Most sophisticated politicians make sure that they are counted as sympathetic to the aging, but give relatively low priority to the elderly among the constituencies from whom they seek votes. . . .

There is little reason to believe that a phenomenon termed "senior power" will significantly increase the proportion of the budget devoted to the aging, or redirect that portion of the budget toward solving the problems of the severely disadvantaged aged. Whatever senior power exists is held by organizations that cannot swing decisive voting blocs. And with the exception of the Gray Panthers, none of the organizations even seek radical change in policies toward the aging.

If anything, the widespread but inaccurate image of senior power may lead most Americans to believe that an imaginary political force of older persons has obtained all that is needed, perhaps more than a fair share, of public resources for the aging. As a consequence, those older persons who are helplessly subject to severe deprivations will not be likely to receive significant attention from our government because they will be hidden within the image of an artificially constructed constituency termed "the aging."

Change our style of policy politics?   Neither senior power nor anything else is forcing us to spend $112 billion on the aging, or to do so with only limited success. Nor will the increasing numbers and proportions of older persons in the decades ahead force us to spend 40% of the federal budget on the elderly in the early years of the twenty-first century. Our current policies reflect our current manner of conducting public business; our future policies will reflect what we choose to do between now and then. . . .

It may very well be that our political leaders are relatively free to mold the economics of aging in whatever directions and fashions that they choose. The conventional wisdom implies that politicians dare not be against the aging, but also that they dare not try to redistribute adequate income to the poor aging. The truth is that no one really tried to defy these assumptions in recent decades. The safe, incremental courses of action have predominated in policies on income and security, health, and social services. This safe style may account for why we are spending so much on intervention policies for the aging and others, but having only limited success.

Certainly there is no reason to feel shackled by projections regarding the costs of programs for the aging over the next few decades. The costs are not fixed, and neither are the resources to support them, because the structures of our current taxing and spending policies are not immutable. Moreover, whatever expenditures we decide to allocate for the aging, even without drastic increases, can be used in a fashion that is much better focused on solving the problems of the severely disadvantaged elderly.

Whether we will exploit these opportunities for change depends upon the willingness of political leaders to transcend the conventional style of conducting the public policy business of the United States. To be sure, there are some risks in discarding safe and familiar routines and in facing unknown consequences. But presumably it is the willingness to take such risks that characterizes those who would be leaders.

Editor's Bridging Comment: On Cost-Benefit Ratios

One of the ways in which program benefits may be enhanced within limited budgets is to increase the number of participants. Much of the overhead cost is inflexible; utilities, staff, rent are quite fixed expenses. In, for example, a nutrition program, the cost of the food is far from the major expense (which is personnel), and the program can reach more people with a small increase in expense. There are, however, problems in mass programs and in programs that show great success rates. Many such programs handle large numbers and achieve great success by "creaming," that is, filling the client slots with those who require less service or are most likely to improve with a small amount of service. The following paper by Tobin and Thompson (1975) shows that numbers aren't everything; indeed, they may merely indicate that the agency is following the path of least resistance, failing to serve the neediest, and generally following the path noted by Binstock: "to them that have shall be given and to them that have not shall be taken the little that they have."

The "Countability" Paradox of Social Programs

S. Tobin and D. Thompson

Purpose. Human benefit—and not "countability"—should be the criterion of professional accountability. The number of participants is too often misleading, and larger numbers of participants may be associated with less personal benefit than when there are fewer participants.

The Study

This paradox—where less participation is associated with more potential benefit—was illustrated in a study of nutrition programs in low-income urban public housing sites. Following conventional wisdom we classified nutrition programs as successful when participation was high and as unsuccessful when participation was low. In addition to the number of participants, four additional criteria were used to select successful programs. These were: participation in other planned activities at housing sites; a positive group identification among participants; involvement in the planning and operation of the nutrition program; and efficient administrative and supervisory practices. By using these five criteria, two successful and two non-successful programs were selected. Within each pair, one program was in a housing site where black elderly lived and the other where white elderly lived. The four nutrition programs selected were among thirty-one operated by a city agency responsible for the planning and development of services for older people.

Organizational Considerations

The four programs were housed in sites that had remarkably similar resident populations being alike on age, sex distribution, income level, and so forth. Each was a five-day-a-week luncheon program where the charge for meals was nominal (45¢, 65¢, or 85¢, depending upon income level). All had a staff of two group workers who also had responsibility for other nutrition programs and elderly aides who served the meals and performed clerical tasks. Socializing among participants was facilitated by these staff and by staff of the host agency.

The average daily attendance was 36 in successful programs and 22 in unsuccessful programs. These numbers represent about 1 of 20 of the resident population at each site (5.2% overall, 4.9% in successful and 5.6% in unsuccessful programs) because the successful programs were in sites that housed larger numbers of residents (about 800 compared to less than 400). As expected, organizational analysis revealed that the successful programs were located at sites which had more social programs, where staff members had warmer and more efficient relationships and where the aides were more flexible and accepting of program participants and other staff members.

Individual Characteristics

We interviewed 10 participants in each program, as well as 10 non-participants who lived at the site (5 who dropped out and 5 who never participated). Of the 80 respondents, 56 were female and 24 were male. All were 65 or over. The average age was 73 and the average income $1914. All had lived at the site for at least one year and were sufficiently lucid to respond to our one to one-and-one-half hour interview.

The attitudes of participants reflected the difference between the two types of programs: participants in unsuccessful programs were less enthusiastic regarding their nutrition programs. Participants in successful and unsuccessful programs differed in other ways as well. . . .

. . . [P]articipants at unsuccessful sites were in poorer health, had lower feelings of well being and less daily activity than non-participants at unsuccessful sites and participants at successful sites were in better health, had greater feelings of well being and more daily activity than non-participants at the site. Given that participants in both types of programs represent similar percentages of their resident populations at the sites, and also that the populations are similar on so many identifying characteristics, it is obvious that participants in successful programs were the better, if not the best, functioning members of their population and that participants in unsuccessful programs were the less adequate, if not the least adequate, members of their population. It was not surprising, therefore, that the interviewer's rating of overall functioning confirmed that the participants in successful programs were functioning far better than non-participants ($p = .009$) whereas participants in unsuccessful programs were judged to be functioning far worse than non-participants ($p = .01$).

These several differences between participants and non-participants were also in evidence when contrasts were made separately between the successful and the unsuccessful programs in black sites and in white sites. There were, however, some interesting differences and similarities between respondents at black and at white sites. Whereas they were alike on morale, functional health, family relationships, dining habits and the interviewer's judgment of overall functioning, blacks had more involvement in organizations, religious groups, and in interpersonal relations. In addition, in successful programs, black participants were markedly different from black non-participants and decidedly more different than were white participants from non-participants. To be specific, black participants in successful programs not only had significantly higher morale, better health, more daily activity, and higher ratings of overall functioning than non-participants, but they also had more organization and interpersonal involvement and were of a somewhat higher socioeconomic class.

At both black and white sites, differences between groups served in successful and unsuccessful programs were also reflected in what participants particularly liked about the program. Most liked by participants in successful programs was the company of other people whereas most liked by participants in unsuccessful programs was having their meals prepared for them. Ill and tending to be depressed, this latter group appreciated the meal itself. Social activities were clearly less important to them than the maintenance of deteriorating physical capacities through various forms of nutrition and health assistance. Curiously enough, participants in successful programs also did not feel that group activity should be provided by nutrition program staffs. Obviously they were already busily occupied in a range of activities.

Discussion

These analyses revealed, therefore, that the two unsuccessful programs were serving a group more in need of social and health services. Less successful programs clearly reached the most needy older people housed at the site. For these older people, the nutrition program was a singular experience in their otherwise rather empty lives.

For participants in successful programs, on the other hand, the program apparently was only one more activity among a variety of activities in which they engaged at the site. Apparently the presence in large numbers of these healthy, high morale, and socially active elderly people limited the participation of others who may have reaped more benefit from the nutrition programs. It seems that in successful programs a small cadre of more vigorous elderly tended to monopolize the program, excluding more needy elderly through subtle and often not so subtle pressures. The staff, in turn, who received more gratification from interaction with these less needy elderly, supported the group process. Apparently the rewards were not for recruiting the more needy to the program, nor for meeting the social and psychological needs of the most needy. Rather, the rewards were for increasing the numbers of participants and maintaining an efficient organization. Efficient they were! They had esprit de corps and their clients had a group identity, as well as being enthusiastic regarding the program. Would they, however, have been as efficient if their clientele were the more needy?

Conclusion

Increasing the count in a program should be secondary to the type of clientele served. Reaching out for the more needy client, however, is only the first step. There must also be a program that meets their needs. It is ironic that in seemingly successful programs, those with less need participated in larger numbers to the likely exclusion of those with more need, whereas in seemingly unsuccessful programs those with more need came in fewer numbers, but because of their very needs could have received the most benefit.

Editor's Comment: On Spawning Social Problem Monsters

Nutrition programs may not be the greatest need of older people. But are mass feeding programs the best answer to that problem? What would have happened if many middle-aged and older house-wives were subsidized to provide hot meals for a few aged living in their immediate vicinity? The capital outlay for stoves, double sinks, meeting health code standards, purchase of dishes, cutlery, and linen could have been avoided and the timid, withdrawn, asocial aged might have more easily been attracted to a much less costly program. Was there prior research to learn about older persons' preference for sociality and education separate from or integrated with nutrition programs? I know that in the personal care homes that dot the Dutch landscape, residents prefer to take their meals in their rooms and to reserve sociality for coffee hours. Or perhaps their caretakers and advocates have only made a different decision for them.

As E. Cohen (1978) has pointed out, we (with the best of intentions) succeed in spawning social-problem monsters—penitentiaries that produce Ph.D.s in crime, a juvenile justice system that succeeds in not much more than incarcerating children without any constitutional guarantees, and similar social innova-tions. One of the recent such backfiring innovations is the deinstitu-tionalization of elderly mental patients. Surely burnt-out schiz-ophrenics and mildly senile older people are no danger to others and, with some community support, need not be locked up in custodially oriented, large state hospitals. Several court decisions by wise and humane judges have established that people who cannot benefit from further treatment and are not dangerous or suicidal may not be incarcerated in mental hospitals. But there was insuffi-cient planning (and financing) to prepare the communities to receive these patients. It was to the states' benefit to have as many patients out of the hospitals as soon as possible for them to live on Federal Supplemental Security Income rather than at state expense and so began the appalling sequence of events described by Donahue (1978). Many patients were reinstitutionalized into nursing homes—that is, smaller institutions lacking in psychiatric care, P.X.s, recreational facilities, films, and other amenities that made the better hospitals more than snake pits. Others ended up in

boarding "homes" and welfare hotels, often unsupervised and un-
licensed, subject to no control, that made the usual mental hospital
seem a country club by contrast. Many wander around "their"
communities in a dazed state, easy marks for any minimally enter-
prising crook. There is literally no place for large numbers of less
than violent people for whom there is no known treatment (who may
not, therefore, be accepted in mental hospitals), who cannot get into
nursing homes, because their behavior is unacceptable (they may
occasionally or more often, fight, scream, curse, and/or throw their
feces around) to nursing and boarding homes, and who absolutely
cannot live in the community. If even nursing homes won't take
them, who can put up with them other than mental hospitals?

This resettlement program might have worked, if it had
evolved more slowly, been properly funded to provide communities
with sufficient resources, and if it had been recognized that some
people need permanent institutional living. For a full description of
this particular monster see Donahue (1978).

Many programs have built-in catch-22s similar to the program
described. That particular catch-22 is that some very deteriorated
people cannot possibly live outside a mental hospital yet cannot be
admitted because they can't be treated, due to the state of the art of
medicine. Another is the catch-22 in home care programs.

To be eligibile, a patient, after a stay in the hospital of at least
three days, must require some element of home *nursing* care, along
with the other required "home helps," such as homemaker service,
help with heavy cleaning, meals-on-wheels, and so on. The patient,
while requiring some nursing service, must be well enough to
perform activities of daily living unaided, yet be too ill or disabled to
get to a physician or clinic. So few people can qualify that home care
services of all kind, including home nursing, account for only 2% of
medicare expenditures (U.S. DHEW, Health Care Financing
Administration, 1978).

Editor's Bridging Comment: The Myth
of the Progressive Income Tax

Another heresy is the problem of proper tax policy. It has long been
a matter of faith among all "right-thinking" people that a progressive
tax structure (that is, one in which the rich pay higher proportions of

their income in taxes than do the poor) is desirable. Yet Wilensky (1978) suggests otherwise. In view of the statistics cited earlier by Binstock (1978), that a fourth of the federal budget, over $100 billion a year, is devoted to programs "for the aged," it behooves us to ponder the novel argument he presents.

The Politics of Taxation: America in World Perspective

H. Wilensky

Every politician knows that taxes cannot be separated from their purpose—spending.

In the 1966 California gubernatorial race, Ronald Reagan sounded the theme that has dominated political rhetoric ever since: taxes are too high, Washington bureaucrats waste money, the man in the middle is being squeezed, and—except for defense—we should cut spending.

After four years in office, with taxes rising and welfare costs soaring, Governor Reagan won reelection on the same slogans: "We are fighting the big spending politicians who advocate a welfare state, the welfare bureaucrats whose jobs depend on expanding the welfare system, and the cadres of professional poor who have adopted welfare as a way of life." George Wallace and Richard Nixon joined the chorus; and by the mid-seventies, candidates Ford and Carter vied with one another for first prize as fiscal conservatives.

Thus was the stage set for the 1978 California tax revolt.

Low Taxes, Lean Spending, Big Backlash

Is our social spending out of line? Compared to other countries, is our tax burden heavy?

The answer is plain: the United States is low in both total taxing and in public spending for social programs. For instance, in relation to gross national product, our spending on Social Security, including aid to the handicapped and the poor, puts us in the lowest third among the nineteen richest democracies. Like Japan, Australia, New Zealand, and Switzerland, we are "welfare-state laggards."

Despite our relatively low total tax burden and relatively meager public programs of health and welfare, what we spend produces an unparalleled political fuss. We move toward the welfare state, but we do it with ill grace, carping and complaining all the way.

"Tax-Welfare Backlash" Abroad

We can explain political uproar in the United States only by comparing other countries.

Surprisingly tax-welfare backlash successes appear among welfare state leaders (Denmark, by 1973 the top spender in the world), middle-rank spenders (Finland, the United Kingdom), and laggards (Switzerland). Apparently, spending that is profligate or lean, taxing that is heavy or light, treatment of the poor that is generous or stingy—all these have little to do with political reaction.

For instance, lean-spending United States and lavish-spending Denmark both produced tax rebellions. Denmark's new "Progress Party," led by tax lawyer Mogens Glistrup, emerged as the second largest parliamentary party in December 1973 when Glistrup advocated:

(1)   Abolishing the income tax by 1980 and burning all papers in the revenue office;

(2)   Wiping out what he called the self-aggrandizing government bureaucracy;

(3)   Abolishing the welfare system and substituting "social guards" in each local community—practical men such as doctors and businessmen who, within a strict budget and with no red tape, would say yes or no to welfare applicants;

(4)   Cutting the pensions of remaining public employees.

Tax Strategies and Social Spending

To put the American and Danish experience in perspective, we can look at the big spenders who have been developing civilized welfare states with relatively little political uproar: countries as diverse as Sweden, Austria, Netherlands, Belgium, and Germany.

The first lesson is that although all modern countries share the spending- taxing explosion, in the calmer big-spending welfare states, the costs of health, welfare, and education rose more smoothly and less visibly, unaccompanied by disruptive rates of unemployment as they were in the United States and Denmark.

Second and more important, the squeeze in disposable income due to rising prices and government expenditures creates most tax resistance in countries that rely too much on painfully visible taxes, especially income taxes and property taxes on households. By "painfully visible," I mean taxes taken directly in one or two big bites from taxpayers who believe that they will not receive direct benefits in line with contributions (social security payroll taxes are moderately visible, but most citizens connect the tax with specific future benefits).

Included in the visible-tax club during the 1960's and early 1970's were such welfare laggards as the United States, Canada, Switzerland, and such middle-rank spenders as the United Kingdom, Finland, and (in the 1960's) Denmark—countries where backlash voting has been prominent.

Although the justification for income taxes in Denmark and the United States alike is "tax the rich, help the poor," the outcome is certain political trouble with no relationship to equality. The United States achieved little income redistribution because our spending has been both lean and hostile to the non-aged poor; Denmark achieved much because its programs have been generous to all, especially to the less privileged. Yet both saw the rise of not only their income taxes but also successful protest candidates, champions of the middle majority.

Contrast the countries with expensive programs, but relatively little tax backlash. They avoid heavy reliance on income and property taxes. Instead, they finance their social programs mainly through indirect taxes such as sales taxes, plus social security contributions of employers and employees.

In December 1977, the U.S. Congress voted to increase social security taxes gradually from 12.1% to 15.3% of taxable pay by 1990. That includes employer and employee contributions and a levy for Medicare.

Many Congressmen, frightened by the apparent protest of their constituents, said, "Let's shift all or some of the increase to general federal revenues." But in the United States, the core of general revenues is the income tax—far more provocative than social insurance contributions.

The myth that we have reached the upper limit of taxation for social programs can be put in perspective by German experience. In 1961, German payroll tax rates for social insurance reached 22.3%, counting employer and employee contributions. A common theme in German public discourse was "people would not tolerate further increases," but by 1973 payroll taxes for health insurance and pensions had climbed to more than 27%—with hardly any political fuss. As our population gets older, we will be forced to follow the German example.

Should taxes be visible?   Traditionally, conservatives have abhorred high taxes, especially progressive income taxes. Yet, if I were a conservative and believed the push for economic equality has gone far enough; if I also believed the welfare state impoverishes the professional and middle classes and rewards the idle and improvident, that "confiscatory taxation" is undermining our economic freedoms while expenditures by "big government" are making everyone a dependent client of the state—if I believed all that, I would break with conservative tradition and advocate a big increase in property taxes on households and in income taxes, the more progressive the better.

Sharply increasing the most painfully visible taxes would provoke such a political fuss that no incumbent big spender would last. Candidates who work the tax-welfare backlash would be successful: they would exercise real power with a mass base.

If, instead, I were a liberal and believed taxes buy civilization, and social spending for health, education, and welfare produces a more humane and just society; if I also believed that a strong government is needed to curb the power of private groups and assure individual security—if I believed all that I would

1. advocate a five-year plan for increasing sales taxes as well as social security taxes on payrolls;

2. gradually phase in a European-style federal value-added tax (tax each business on the difference between sales to its customers and its purchases from other businesses—i.e., its value added);

3. recognize that governments cannot expand cash benefits and social services without increasing the tax take;

4. accept the need for tax balance. I would avoid too much reliance on what surveys show are the most unpopular taxes—property taxes on households and personal income taxes.

Misguided enthusiasm for painfully visible taxes will keep the country in turmoil without producing enough revenue to meet citizen demands.

Editor's Comment

Alternatives to some special programs for the aged may well be explored. Less obtrusive tax schemes, plus programs that allow the aged and other groups to combine their forces for programs that benefit them all might be politically more palatable than special programs for special groups. We might raise some questions about the growing Balkanization of American politics on the basis of class and ethnicity, with each group struggling for its allocation of resources and attempt to secure services to meet the needs of all needy groups, for example, some feasible national health insurance scheme rather than incremental increases in Medicare and/or minimum income provisions for all instead of Supplemental Security Income provisions for some. It is politically more astute to make coalitions than for each group to "be in business for itself."

Recommended Readings

Kammerman, S. and Kahn, A. *Not for the Poor Alone: European Social Services.* Philadelphia: Temple University Press, 1975.

Neugarten, B. and Havighurst, R. *Social Policy, Social Ethics and the Aging Society.* Washington, D.C.: National Science Foundation, 1976.

———. *Extending the Human Life Span: Social Policy and Social Ethics.* Washington, D.C.: National Science Foundation, 1977.

Wershow, H. "Setting Priorities in Health and Welfare Services." *Health and Social Work* l(1977):6–24.

———. "The Outer Limits of the Welfare State: Discrimination, Racism and Their Effect on Human Services." *Aging and Human Development* 10 (1979–1980):63–75.

10

Organic Brain Syndrome: A Case Study of Wishful Formulation of Social Policy in Caring for the Aged

*First you forget names, then you forget faces, then you forget to pull
your zipper up, then you forget to pull your zipper down.*
Leo Rosenberg, quoted in Lawrence J. Peter,
Peter's Principles: Ideas for our Time.

Editor's Introduction

The contents of this chapter are drawn from several sources. Much
are various excerpts from a British journal, *Age and Ageing,* which
devoted a special supplement (Anderson and Carlton-Ashton, 1977)
to "Brain Failure in the Aged." Arie, in a short excerpt from that
volume, notes the vigor with which gerontologists attempt to avoid
dealing with that problem, which Wershow (1977c) shows is overwhelming. The impact of organic brain syndrome (OBS) on the
family is noted by Brocklehurst (1977) who utilizes, in a paper from
the *Age and Ageing* volume, some data from the immediate postwar
period to show that this problem has not changed. The advisability
of vigorous treatment of those with advanced OBS is questioned by
another British observer (Anonymous, 1977). We end with a discussion of a problem raised in the *Age and Ageing* symposium on a
problem rarely discussed in the United States, of segregating those
with OBS from other institutionalized aged versus integrating them
in institutions serving other chronically ill aged.

Manifestations of chronic Organic Brain Syndrome (OBS) occur
in about 3–4% of those over 65 (Brocklehurst, 1977), but the preva-

lence increases with advancing age; an as yet unknown proportion of those age 75 and up suffer from this condition. Nice gerontologists don't talk about OBS. As a British observer noted:

> A head-on approach to this massive challenge to all health services is often frustrated by diversionary attacks on two fronts; one is from the sociologists who attempt to explain away dementia so as to make it vanish by postulating a primacy to environmental factors; the other comes from our own profession [medicine], which sometimes verges on diagnosing away dementia. The suggestion is that if one is clever enough, one will find that they are all in fact hypothyroid, depressed, or something else. The menace of both these approaches is that they each have a degree of truth in them, but they may ultimately detract from an effective approach to this problem on which we should all be embarked. (discussion by Arie following Brocklehurst, 1977)

When the subject of OBS was raised in the following paper (Wershow, 1977c), the editor of *The Gerontologist* noted that it was high time to take this unseen plague out of the closet, recognize its epidemic proportions among the very old, its leading to institutionalization and irresistible progressivity (E. Cohen, 1977). He described the note that follows as harsh and one of the most controversial pieces ever published in *The Gerontologist*.

Reality Orientation for Gerontologists—Some Thoughts about Senility

H. Wershow

Introduction

This paper had its genesis in the author's reaction to the violent emotions engendered by a discussion of "senility" which took place in Jerusalem in June, 1975 at a pre-Congress colloquium of the European Social Research Committee of the International Association of Gerontology. Most of the participants in that colloquium refused to accept the fact that, for the present and forseeable future, there will remain a large number of persons suffering from chronic organic brain syndrome (OBS), an irreversible disorder of learning and memory. Now that death and dying are more freely discussed, it is obvious that senile dementia, or chronic OBS, and the problems it presents remains a taboo topic. Only optimistic approaches to the problems are admitted into professional consideration. Wherever possible, misleading analogies are presented, so that the differences between OBS and reversible pathologies are obscured and obfuscated. Social scientists try to explain away OBS with disengagement and labeling theory. Claims are made that old people develop OBS—become senile, in the same way that college students develop depressive symptoms which may mimic the effects of OBS, in experimental situations in which the students are constantly belittled and denigrated. In the aged as in younger people, depressive reactions may occur, which often present some similarities to OBS. It is also true that some older persons may tend to withdraw from activity and personal relationships in the absence of senility and that behavioral and emotional problems in the aged are too often needlessly attributed to OBS. But the reality of this common pathology cannot be denied. Denial may be a functional defense mechanism in the face of impossible adversity in patients and their families. It is an indefensible reaction in a professional and scientific community. However discouraging, even frightening, the problem of senility may be, its implications must be faced squarely and dealt with. It should be recognized that much of what we practice and advocate in the psychosocial area may be inappropriate in the treatment of OBS. So far, we have been markedly unsuccessful in reversing OBS by either organic or sociopsychological therapies. Most factors implicated in the genesis of OBS are not readily amenable to prophylactic intervention, e.g., alcoholism and atherosclerosis. However, psychological and toxic states leading to acute OBS are often treatable. There is evidence that various psychological manipulations and prosthetic environments may make it possible for some patients to function with less stress to themselves and others (Goldfarb, 1956; Gurian and Scherl, 1972; Kramer and Kramer, 1966, 1967). In any case, all cases of OBS should be thoroughly worked up by a competent, multidisciplinary team. . . .

In this paper, we will define the problem, estimate its growing dimensions, and discuss some implications of that growth. Full descriptions and discussion of chronic OBS can be found in Goldfarb (1974), Sandok (1975), and Wells (1972). For the purposes of this discussion it is sufficient to state that OBS is inexorably progressive, that it progresses from increasing cognitive and judgmental disability to eventual (if death does not intervene) complete helplessness, total dependency, loss of sphincter control, in short, functioning at no more than a vegetative level. The proportion of sufferers increases with age to an unknown but high proportion at age 85 and older. Fifteen to 30% is not an uncommon estimate.

Current and Future Prevalence of OBS

OBS of the irreversible type is epidemic in nursing homes and similar institutions in the USA and elsewhere in the developed world. Studies indicate that at least 60–80% (Wershow, 1977b) of the elderly patients in nursing homes and up to 85% (Goldfarb, 1962) of first admissions to protected settings suffer from irreversible OBS. More conservative estimates, perhaps resulting from stricter criteria, of 50–60% from Gregory (1970) and Stotsky (1966) are confirmed by the estimates of Anderson (1977), Vital Health Statistics (VHS) (1973), and Social Security Administration (SSA) (U.S., Department of Health, Education and Welfare, 1974). SSA (1974) survey of nursing and homes for the aged (which latter contain fewer advanced OBS) informs us that 45% of the residents were "occasionally and usually confused" and 59% were unable to manage their income and spending money. VHS (1973) estimates 56.4% of residents of nursing homes as senile to moderate or severe degrees. We will accept a conservative estimate that 50% of the patients in nursing homes suffer from irreversible OBS, or about 500,000 individuals. VHS (1973) estimates that 1.3% of the civilian noninstitutionalized elderly population (65+) is senile (including advanced) or 260,000 individuals which, added to the institutional population, yields a bit over 750,000 senile people in the USA today (plus some 60,000 in mental hospitals).

This estimate is of the same order of magnitude as are surveys of the aged population in other technologically advanced societies. . . . However, the truly frightening dimensions of the problem of OBS are only beginning to emerge. The greatest proportional growth in the aged population is the rapid increase in *older* old people, i.e., those over 75 and 80 years of age.

> The older population itself is aging and is expected to continue to age. The proportion of 65 to 69 of the group 65 and over is getting smaller, while the proportion 75 and over is getting larger, and this trend is expected to continue at least to the end of the century. In 1900 the proportion over 75 was 29%. By 1970 this proportion has risen to 38%. By the year 2000, we may expect about 43% of the 65-and-over group to fall into the 75-and-over group (Siegel, 1974).

Forty-three percent of the 28,850,000 aged 65+ in the year 2000 would mean 12,400,000 individuals aged 75+. These estimates are not unreasonable. Even in 1969, and today, the average USA white male aged 65 can expect to live to age 78 and the female to age 81.6 (Siegel, 1974). Considerable numbers, especially females, even now survive well into their 80s.

The Cost of Care of OBS Patients

Let us look ahead to the implications of that increase in the *older* elderly. Let us conservatively assume, despite their proportionate increase in the population aged 65+, that the proportion institutionalized of those aged 75+ will remain the same as today, about 14–15% (Anderson, 1976). That estimate would yield about 1,600,000 patients aged 75+ in nursing homes and similar institutions, about 66% more than the total current population aged 65+ so institutionalized. Let us make some additional far from "worst-case" assumptions: that no more than 60% of these patients will have OBS despite their advanced age (or one million persons), a modest estimate but double the number of those aged 65+ currently institutionalized with OBS. It is also certain that the cost of their care will be considerably more than three times the current expenditure of $3,000/patient/year, cited by SSA (1974). The national average cost of nursing home care can very easily rise to $10,000/patient/year in constant dollars by the year 2000, due to rapidly rising costs of construction, maintenance, interest, labor, and automation of care. It is also quite possible that medical advances may make it possible to double the institutional life-span of nursing home patients (that life-span is currently measured in no more than days or weeks for most) (Kastenbaum and Candy, 1973; Palmore, 1976b; Wershow, 1976); the number of nursing home patients will then double beyond the projection of one million. With two million patients, we arrive at the sum of twenty billion dollars a year for merely the room, board, and nursing components of care. Physicians' services, drugs, dental, optical, podiatric care, intercurrent acute hospitalization and surgery, and all other expenses are excluded from this calculation. Yet this sum for the nursing care of those institutionalized aged 75+ suffering from chronic OBS will amount to 80% of the total current USA medical care expenditure for all aged 65+. If the cost of care or the length of stay of patients in nursing homes increases markedly, this estimate may increase astronomically. Indeed, the cost of nursing home care in New York is today commonly estimated to be $20,000/patient/year. The projections made herein are, therefore, quite conservative.

Policy Considerations

We take issue with those "advocates" for the aged who set no priorities but who call for more and more and more of better and better (Neugarten, 1975). The aged are not an affluent group in the USA, but they do receive a share of health and welfare expenditures at least proportional to their numbers, though not sufficient to meet their needs. The aged receive the major share of funds expended by such massive programs as Social Security, Supplemental Security Income, veterans' aid, Medicare, and Medicaid. Programs for the aged in the USA are not luxurious, nor even adequate, but the aged are not discriminated against in the distribution of public resources. . . .

We do suggest that we abandon our fantasies of therapeutic omnipotence, that we cease the terribly expensive and useless therapies vigorously conducted over long periods which always turn out to be no more than minimal in their effects. These efforts should clearly be labeled as experimental and limited to a few carefully selected centers, as are trials of new drugs. To tout them as useful and to apply them indiscriminately and widely leads to disaster (Gubrium and Ksander, 1975). Whatever success has been achieved is rendered problematic in that no research, to our knowledge, has limited its experimental subjects to those with unequivocal evidence of demonstrated brain atrophy. . . . We seriously question any research that is not thus limited, recognizing that:

> While isolated instances do occur in which there is poor correlation between psychological dysfunction and brain pathology, these are the exceptions. . . . In general, all recent studies have demonstrated a close correlation between degrees of social and psychological dysfunction and severity of brain pathology (Wells, 1972).

The most sophisticated research to date has been conducted by the Philadelphia Geriatric Center (PGC) (Brody et al., 1971, 1973, 1974; Kleban et al., 1975, 1976). Most other studies are conducted among younger target populations of functionally disturbed or at best, a mixed bag of neurological and psychiatric defects and in institutions which lack the extensive treatment resources of PGC. Examples of the more usual research can be seen in Goldstein and Shelly (1975) and Harris and Ivory (1976). Goldstein and Shelly's oldest patient was 62 and mean age of the "old" subject group was 51.3. But these authors did attempt to eliminate subjects with lateralized or focal lesions and focus on those with diffuse brain lesions, based on evidence that included such diagnostic tests as angiography and brain scans. Harris and Ivory's subjects' mean age was 66.6, with an age range of 36 to 81 and a mixed diagnostic bag of modally paretics, chronic and organic brain syndromes, and mentally deficient. Over 60 of the latter's 96 subjects suffered a variety of other diagnoses; the major common factor, we suspect, was less their medical diagnoses than a mean hospitalization duration of over 20 years.

The PGC data focused sharply on *old* people, mean age over 81 and Kahn Goldfarb Mental Status Questionnaire (MSQ) (1960) mean scores of 3.2 at the onset of the 3-year study, plus a psychiatric-neurological examination confirming the diagnosis of moderate to severe OBS. Even this relatively low level of functioning does not approach the deficits attained by our unselected (for OBS) sample of nursing home patients of whom over 75% could not answer one question on the MSQ in proprietary homes in Alabama (Wershow, 1977b). It should be made clear that the objective of the PGC long-term study was *not to reverse the effects of OBS*, but rather to treat "excess disability," i.e., the gap between actual and potential functioning in many spheres, as determined by a multidisciplinary team in what is generally recognized as an institution with one of the most progressive treatment programs in this country, if not the world. The treatment program is not described, except to note that it was intensive, individualized, and concentrated. Having personal knowledge of the PGC, we freely acknowledge that it was of heroic dimensions. Yet the result of a whole year of intensive treatment is less than modest. Only 16% of the excess disability variance between experimental and control groups (the latter receiving the usual level of PGC treatment) was due to the experimental variable. Most of the variance is explained by initial characteristics of the subjects; those who profited the most were those relatively younger subjects with greater intersocial competence, interpersonal sensitivity, ability to engage in activity and be self-sufficient, relative to the abilities of others in this group, which the PGC people like to characterize as "mentally frail." Improvements were greatest in the areas of family relationships and individualized activities, to a lesser extent in self-care and self-sufficiency. We are not told the extent to which this first improvement resulted from counseling with family members other than the patient. The rest were, almost by definition of "excess disability," the result of individual design of activities within the scope of ability of patients whose capabilities and limitations became better known to staff as a result of the experiment. Is treatment of "excess disability" much more than explication of what passes unmentioned in most studies as placebo effect?

Also, it is necessary to differentiate between statistical and clinical significance. A datum may be statistically significant, though of a magnitude insufficient to make much difference in the subjects' functioning, even in the prosthetic environment of PGC. About all the study showed was that those younger, initially less damaged subjects functioned in that environment better than those with more severe brain damage throughout the three year period. The only two cases presented in the series of papers deal with what seems to be emotional overlay added to the intellectual deficit of relatively intact subjects. We hope that the PGC group continues its work in this area, but adds a more definitive diagnosis of OBS by use of methods such as dynamic brain scan and/or computerized transaxial tomography to establish neuroanatomical deficits. Incidentally and not surprisingly, the year of intensive treatment had no effect on the subjects two years later; the pre-morbid personality and initial level of functioning were the relevant factors. This is not meant to denigrate the PGC studies, which demonstrate that therapeutic nihilism is unwarranted. Therapeutic omnipotence is equally unwarranted.

It is time that we accept the reality that brain cells, once destroyed, do not regenerate. We must recognize that special institutions for the severely damaged senile dements require few mental-psychological therapies. These patients need large amounts of nursing care so that they may die with relative dignity and in as much comfort as society can afford them. That we can do anything more to decrease their suffering and to increase their pleasure is, at best, highly questionable if not totally illusory. It is also questionable that we "help" anyone by extensive provision of home care and community support systems to families of these severely senile patients. No one should be made to feel guilty (the current hue and cry against insitutional care does just that) for their "failure" to keep patients with advanced chronic OBS at home. Home care with adequate supports may be ideal for some, but reasonable alternatives to twenty-four hour professional care do not exist for this group. . . .

Research, with the few exceptions noted, should be directed into channels more productive than social-psychological therapies, into mundane areas which few deign to investigate. We need to engineer mechanical devices that make it easier to keep patients clean and comfortable, such as a bed that can dispose of products of incontinence without restraining a patient and without the use of infection-creating catheters. We need to find ways to best supervise and give emotional support to the less trained aides, LPNs, and others who bear the brunt of caring for these patients, surely one of the least rewarding jobs imaginable. We need to train and place in these institutions good geriatric nurse-practitioners, who need precisely that measure of care that can best be offered by a good nurse practitioner. We must realize that for every person, at some time, the moment arrives when *our* need to "do something" is inappropriate, even grotesque. Solomon may have been correct, 2300 years ago, when he said in Ecclesiastes (11:1–3):

> To everything there is a season, and a time to
> every purpose under the heaven;
> A time to be born and a time to die;
> A time to plant and a time to up-root that which
> is planted.

Editor's Comment: Controversy around Wershow Paper*

Though the above paper very carefully (it seemed to us) stated both that only a small percentage of the aged, even of the very old, become demented and that much of what passes as and is mistakenly diagnosed as chronic OBS is reversible, the predictable responses were accusations of "stereotyping" (Hellebrandt, 1978; G. Cohen, 1978; Armstrong, 1978), "the effect of absence of environmental or motivational stimuli in the institutional setting . . . the lack of treatment" (Settin, 1978, p. 71), denial that end-stage OBS exists in the cruel and painful (to family and friends perhaps more than to the dement) form described. Armstrong (1978) proclaims that end-stage patients "attend programs almost daily . . . have romances . . . enjoy old films from the '30s . . . participate in painting, crafts" (p. 315), and so on, and Hellebrandt (1978) tells us they tell and listen to stories (but note only those "capable of verbalizations") and readings from the newspaper. She mentioned in passing the existence of another division of the institution she describes "with hospital beds and restraining chairs." All comments about the "Reality Orienta-tion" paper studiously ignore problems of the very regressed, vegetative patients we have noted in our paper. Armstrong (1978) claims that they "may have as long as five years, perhaps longer, to live" (p. 315), while Hellebrandt (1978) admits that many "eventual-ly become mute, mindless, and incontinent," but hopes that "some intercurrent infection or complicating chronic degenerative disease terminates life before a vegetative existence ensues" (p. 67). Ignored is the inadvisability of vigorous treatment at this stage, precisely the question raised in our paper, though prayerfully and tentatively, and not without great trepidation. I do teach a course on The Holocaust as well as gerontology.

   Insensitive disclaimers are filed aginst our assertion that we help no one by "extensive provision of home care and community support systems to families of these severely senile patients" (Wer-show, 1977c, p. 151).

   "It is difficult to understand the author's blanket condemnation of community services" (Settin, 1978, p. 71). Another viewpoint is

---

*Short quotations from Hellebrandt, G. Cohen, Armstrong, and Settin are used with the permission of the Gerontological Society.

presented from a British source. Brocklehurst (1977) cites Sheldon's (1947) study of 477 aged in Wolvert-Hampton, England, and comments on the great burdens shouldered by families of those suffering from OBS.

Brain Failure in Old Age: Social Implications

J. Brocklehurst

. . . The most relevant aspect of Sheldon's findings in relation to mental confusion was that of the strain which was shouldered by relatives, who had to care for them. He found that in all, 57 (14.7%) of the old people seen were causing strain on those who looked after them and that in about half of these cases the strain was severe and almost intolerable. This was not always because of mental abnormality but the latter is rated highly among the causes of strain. The following is a typical case:

> A woman in her late 70's suffers from anxiety so that she is terrified of being left alone and at the same time has become increasingly suspicious. Her daughter-in-law who looks after her can get out only for shopping—she never goes out to amusements and had had no relief for nine years, during which time she had to deal with many difficult situations.

In fact in the case of 57 patients who were causing strain, 29% of the relatives found holidays impossible. In 37% of the cases the only time the daughter (or chief carer) was able to go out, was for shopping. In regard to the 7% of cases in which the relatives were under extreme strain, he said that this implied

> a mode of existence which deprived the individual of a normal life and turned her into a drudge . . . there is only one description possible, they are working in a sweated industry. This actually understates the true position for it takes no account of the deep emotional stresses that may be imposed by difficulties of behavior in an old person who may suffer from some degree of mental impairment, and by such possiblities as the surrender of their own chances of normal domesticity.

Twenty-eight years ago Sheldon suggested the need for an increase in short-term or holiday admissions for the relief of relatives' strain.

The importance of relief of relatives' strain in admission of old people to hospital has been underlined by Issacs et al. (1972) in their survey of admissions to geriatric wards, in Glasgow.

Sheldon ends his work with the following statement.

Although the experimental development of hostels for a temporary stay is strongly advocated as a means whereby the family affection may be preserved and at the same time the community may discharge its duty to those of its members who are carrying a disproportionate share of the burden of old age, the facts nevertheless remain that the most urgent need is for more accommodation of the aged on a permanent basis. This is perhaps the greatest single requirement for the welfare of the aged at the present time.

Editor's Comment

Robinson (discussion following Brocklehurst, 1977) adds that:

It is all very well to talk about support at home, but a sizeable proportion of this group can no longer be maintained at home in anything like a civilized fashion. I think that the home for the mentally confused or impaired at least gives us another string to our placement bow to the range of therapeutic possibilities.

The points raised here about the increasing cost of care, projecting greatly increased numbers of patients with chronic OBS and the inapplicability of any treatment to these unfortunate souls, are not the only controversies raging around the care of aged with OBS.

The British experience and philosophy, unlike the American, is not to engage in vigorous efforts to prolong life when the quality of life is poor.

The issues aired above by Sheldon, Brocklehurst and Robinson in *Brain Failure and the Aged* (1977), and in the discussion by Wershow about the exponential rise in cost of care of the ever-growing older and therefore ever more heavily weighted with OBS population are grave indeed. What are we to do with the tremendous projected financial and emotional cost of caring for these untreatable patients? The time may soon arrive, as medical care rises in cost from 8 to 10 to ever higher percentages of the GNP, that we as a society will have to ponder the wisdom of Solomon. Is there "a time to die?" and have we striven too officiously to delay that time beyond reason? We may someday (and perhaps soon) have to consider the wisdom of alternative ways of playing God, either by giving or withholding antibiotics, diuretics, and other treatment from those whose quality of life is diminishing below some point to be determined (by patient, family, physician, or explicit rationing of medical resources?). A British experience, at variance with our usual American practice, follows.

Case Conference:
. . . Strive Officiously to Keep Alive?

Anonymous

Case Report

Mr. A. B. and his family were well known in the county town in which they lived. For the whole of his life he had involved himself deeply in his local community. He was a teacher at a local school where he worked a great deal to organize hobbies, sports, etc., after hours for the children, and did not confine himself to his official duties. He was an active member of the local cricket club and became its secretary for ten years before, in his early 50s, it was recognized that he was suffering from the early signs of a presenile dementia. Over the course of three years this popular, extroverted, active man went through the progressive disintegration of personality which accompanies the dementia. He could never understand or accept the reason for his dismissal from the school as he had no insight into his problem. He went through a period of paranoia and aggressiveness in response to this which seemed quite alien to his temperament. He became upset when his views were not accepted at the cricket club committee, and eventually the right to attend was refused, intensifying his distress. He gradually settled, however, into a contented pattern of life as the dementia became more profound. He was a widower, and fortunately had one widowed daughter living a few houses away, who agreed to come to live in his house to care for him. For about a year he led a peaceful life in this way, pottering in the garden, sitting in the sun, and watching television without comprehension, but some pleasure. He was clearly confused on day-to-day events, could not dress himself, although he valued his appearance, and could not carry out even simple purposeful activities without assistance. He would become confused at meals and when unable to complete a task would appear distressed and cry. He retained his genial personality and enjoyed the presence of visitors although he could not remember their names or who they were, even with quite close friends. It was hard to say whether this was a life of suffering. His daughter felt that he had never fully understood why it was that he had had to leave his school and his cricket club and live a life of relative isolation. She knew that conversation of his past or reminders, such as old photographs, etc., would immediately obviously cause him anguish, with tearfulness and a mood of lethargy and depression which would last for several days. He seemed to bear a burden of a sense of loss which he could not understand.

The Choice for Doctor and Daughter

I had known him as his general practitioner for a year and in that time had witnessed a gradual decline in his capacity to cope with the simple activities of the house. He moved about less, spoke less, and took almost no initiative, although remaining always welcoming and cheerful. He developed 'flu in the early winter and a mild upper respiratory infection which I treated with a five-day course of oxytetracycline. Following this he was never really well and insidiously developed congestive cardiac failure. He appeared in no distress, but was generally weak, unable to get out of bed, and had some orthopnoea so that he was allowed to sleep sitting up. At this point his daughter raised the question of the necessity to treat him other than by measures designed to keep him comfortable. There was no element of self interest in her request. She was a woman of independent means who was clearly devoted to her father and said she would continue the responsiblity of his care for another ten years if necessary. But she felt that his life had lost its dignity and meaning, that he was aware of his disability, and suffered through the inability to understand it, and that he had always stated his fear of being a burden on his family. We agreed to treat him conservatively. We managed the ankle oedema with supportive bandages and propping up the foot of the bed, gave him a mild sedative at night, and arranged for night nurses so that he would never be left unattended. Over a period of three weeks he gradually became weaker, although at no time in distress from dyspnoea or any other obvious discomfort. . . . Over the next weekend the patient suddenly deteriorated, becoming feverish and confused. I attended frequently, monitoring the dose of sedation required to minimize his confusion but not to cause excessive drowsiness. He gradually deteriorated and died within forty-eight hours. His daughter was present almost constantly and felt that her father had had a peaceful and calm end to his life. . . . (pp. 189–190).

Editor's Comment: The Senile—
Integration into the Institution

One of the great problems in the care of the senile is: where to put them? For better or for worse, they can no longer be kept in the state mental hospitals. In these large institutions, there were at least enough sufferers from OBS to segregate the more deteriorated and those whose bizarre conduct disturbs their fellow patients the most. With the forced exit of custodial patients from the state institutions, they have been incorporated into other settings (however ill-equipped to deal with their problems). They must now coexist with the more intellectually aware, comprehending aged, and we know little about the effect of that interaction. What has been the effect of so-called "deinstitutionalization" of the senile aged? How well do they coexist with other patients in their new settings of nursing home, care home or boarding house?

We are unaware of any professional discussion of the problem of separate institutions for the chronic OBS patients versus integrating them into more general institutions. However, the British professional community, here as in other areas of social policy, well ahead of the United States in its planning for and committment to social welfare, is engaged in debate about the merits of ways of caring for sufferers from OBS.

Brocklehurst (1977) raises the question in this manner:

Brain Failure in Old Age: Social Implications

J. Brocklehurst

. . . The practical problem of confused old people in residential care has led to two different forms of management, that of integration in which the confused and the rational live together and that of segregation where special homes are built for the mentally confused old people or in a more limited way special parts of already existing homes are used for their accommodation. Meacher's book *Taken for a Ride* (1972) is a survey of six homes, three falling into each of these two categories. His objective was to discover whether there was justification for the existence of special (or separatist, as he called them) homes and what were the effects both on the confused old people and also on the non-confused and on the staff. He also studied wards in a mental hospital and in a very large former public assistance institution. Altogether 329 old people were interviewed and information sought about their backgrounds. They were also psychologically assessed. Meacher points out that probably one-seventh of people in post-war residential homes are mentally impaired and that the proportion in former workhouses is much higher. The major problem that they pose is that of non-conforming behaviour which is expressed in such things as undressing themselves in public and passing urine in inappropriate places. In comparing a number of physical correlates he found that only incontinence and impaired hearing significantly correlated with the confused. . . .

Perhaps one of the most significant things that Meacher found was some manifestation of confused behaviour in at least 16% of patients in normal homes and in only 58% of those in separatist homes. In other words more than two-fifths of the residents in the special homes for the mentally confused were in no way confused. He found that these homes were used also for the accommodation of those who might be less socially acceptable in ordinary residential homes, either because of their social backgrounds or because of unpleasant habits; indeed many normal people were admitted there because, when a crisis arose and a place had to be found quickly in a residential home, less regard was paid to the distinctions between confusion and non-confusion.

Meacher comes out against separatist homes and his main reason for this (apart from the fact that they are not used properly) is that they tend to pre-judge mental confusion and the attitude of the staff becomes stereotyped towards accepting everything in a patient's behaviour as due to confusion. This leads to an overuse of drugs, to an absence of integrative activities which might retrieve the confused person from his confusion and so to a condemning of those who are admitted to such homes to confirmed and progessive confusion.

It is important to see his argument linked to the fact that he considers a good deal of mental confusion in old people to be socially inspired rather than the result of organic disease. It is on this concept of mental confusion that his thesis seems to be most vulnerable. He does, however, correctly indicate that the doctrine of separatism may have stigmatizing implications and that this may affect the recruitment of staff and discourage the attention of visitors. This is a matter that is familiar to all who practice in the field of geriatric medicine and one to which we will be sympathetic. In some ways the arguments against having separate homes for the mentally confused are the same as the arguments against having special hospitals for geriatric patients. (pp. 33–34)

[There follows an interesting discussion between Professor Brocklehurst and colleagues.]

Dr. Bergmann: Professor Brocklehurst has been very kind and perhaps especially tolerant of the stance taken by Meacher. I would like therefore to have the opportunity of continuing my long-standing quarrel with Meacher. I wonder what he feels about the following things that Meacher has done. Firstly he has confused people with organic psychiatric disorders of the chronic brain failure type with those who are pushed out of handicap institutions, and with those who are the graduate schizophrenics of mental hospitals. He has produced a behaviour scale which compounds all three situations. This is not to say that I do not think that they should be mixed, but he certainly fails to distinguish between them. Secondly he has chosen separatist terms where I think on Professor Brocklehurst's account and certainly on Meacher's account the worst people were put into the worst homes. There is however a model separatist home that was existing, and does exist, in which positive discrimination is given. Here best homes are custom designed, there is night attendance and psychiatric supervision. Certainly in Newcastle we have worked with this model for many years where the patients get a better deal than ordinary residential care and they need it. That includes bringing in services and bringing in community people and occupational therapists to a much greater degree than ordinary residential homes can afford to do. I think the separatist case is a very much better one than perhaps came through, perhaps because Professor Brocklehurst was trying to be more fair minded than I think he should have been. (p. 36)

Professor Brocklehurst: The importance of Meacher's contribution is that it puts a point of view which should make us think very hard. The mere fact that two-fifths of people in the homes that he looked at were not confused and yet that these were homes for mentally confused people, is something important to note; especially when he points out the implications of staff attitudes. That these are often unrecognized is the importance of this thesis. . . .

In the world in which we are living there is no doubt that old people are admitted to special homes for the confused because their behaviour is unacceptable in another home and the matron does not like them. They get moved into this one by an arrangement with the social welfare officer. Similarly if the old man is a tramp and dishevelled he is not seen by a doctor, which is absolutely wrong, but it is the present mechanism. . . . (p. 39)

Dr. Middleton: If one subscribes to the integrated concept rather than the separatist, what does one do with Dr. Bergmann's streakers or the faecal scatterers or the persistent thief of other patients' 'belongings'? I think it is unfair to subject people who are normal intellectually to an existence twenty-four hours a day with this type of individual. Should one have sub-units of perhaps ten residents, an idea that has been suggested by Townsend and others for those requiring residential accommodation? For all of us here when we become old, living in a home is unnatural. The vast majority of old people have been brought up in a nuclear family or ex-tended family. The other point Professor Brocklehurst mentioned is the high number of individuals in institutions in Scandinavia. Those of us who have studied Scandinavia realize this. In Sweden for instance, there are something like six times as many beds for geriatric patients as we have in Britain, and approximately four times as many places in homes for the elderly, and yet, wherever one goes in Sweden one is faced with the problems of long waiting lists and the serious geriatric problem. (p. 39)

Professor Brocklehurst: One can say about Meacher's book, that it forms a good (and controversial) basis for discussion. It brings up many points which are important and which otherwise we might not think about. But I do agree that it is difficult (certainly we imagine it is difficult) for old people in a home to have somebody who is behaving very badly beside them. First of all, Meacher says the residents are very often bothered about other things far more than they are bothered about the old person's behaviour and they take that old person along with them and try to help him and integrate him as much as possible. Secondly there is a danger that we accept such things as faecal scattering and so on as being facts of life when they are not and almost certainly something can be done about them.

Perhaps we ought to think from time to time of the tremendous stress on relatives in keeping some old people at home. Obviously there are very good reasons why most old people should be maintained in the community but it does hide a lot of intolerable stress as Sheldon showed. I think the figure of 7% may well apply today in terms of severe stress on the shoulders of people who have to care for old people. Short-term admissions are necessary and I am sure we could use our accommodation more sensibly. (p. 39)

Dr. Irvine: On the question of mutual tolerance, confused and unconfused patients, there seems to be a conflict of evidence about what people really feel about this. Brocklehurst reports Meacher as showing that there is really a high degree of mutual tolerance and yet I believe the hospital advisory service found that the commonest form of complaint from geriatric wards is patients who are mentally normal finding themselves associating with patients who are not mentally normal. I would also like to pass on a comment for discussion. A very good social worker once told me that he thought the answer to this problem was the length of time the people had been together in a home. If an old lady in a home started off relatively normal but became more confused after she had established relationships with other patients they would carry her along as Meacher described. If, on the other hand, a lady was introduced into a home from scratch with disturbed behaviour she was quite likely to be rejected. (pp. 39–40)

Professor Brocklehurst: These are important matters for us to consider and discuss, and if policy is based on the results of surveys which are mistaken in some of their percepts, then this is sad comment and an important matter to correct. (p. 40)

Editor's Note

This discussion is presented to the American gerontologists to move some of us to undertake studies that may lead to better social policy.

Recommended Readings

Anderson, F. W. and Carlton-Ashton, J. R., eds. "Brain Failure and Old Age." *Age and Ageing* (Supplementary Issue) 6 (1977).

Chiompi, L. and Muller, Ch., eds. *Senile Dementia: Clinical and Therapeutic Aspects*. Bern and Stuttgart: Huber Press, 1968.

Gaitz, C., ed. *Aging and the Brain*. New York: Plenum, 1972.

Goldfarb, A. *Aging and Organic Brain Syndrome*. New York: Health Learning System, 1974.

Gubrium, J. F. and Ksander, M. "On Multiple Realities and Reality Orientation." *Gerontologist* 15 (1975): 142–45. Those interested in seeing how Reality Orientation programs are carried out by untrained subprofessionals are referred to this account, which would be hilarious if it were not so sad.

Sandok, B. A. "Organic Brain Syndromes." In *Comprehensive Textbook of Psychiatry*, vol I, edited by A. M. Friedman, H. L. Kaplan, and B. J. Sadock. Baltimore: Williams and Wilkins, 1975.

11

Are Older People More Likely To Be Victims of Criminals?

We know accurately only when we know little; with knowledge, doubt enters.

Goethe

Editor's Introduction

One of the more prevalent beliefs about the elderly is that they are more often victimized by criminals than other age groups. Two views are here presented; both utilize different aspects of the same data and come to different conclusions. It is most interesting to compare the two papers, to see how preconceptions can lead to selective perception and good will can lead investigators to erroneous conclusions (Wershow, 1963).

The Scope of Victimization of the Elderly

A. Malinchak and D. Wright

"Psychologically, financially, and physically, no group of citizens suffers more painful losses than our Nation's elderly do at the hands of America's criminal predators." (U.S., Congress, House, April 1976). Nevertheless, confusion and doubt exist about the scope of the national problem, stemming largely from three factors:

— Elderly victims often do not report crimes (Hindelang, 1975),

— Law enforcement officials are not aware of the special needs of elderly crime victims, and

— The subject of elderly crime victimization has been approached in a "bandwagon" fashion, rather than in an orderly, interdisciplinary manner, resulting in unreliable data.

As Jack Goldsmith and Noel E. Tomas (1974) reported in an earlier issue of *Aging*, the underreporting of crime by the elderly is a major roadblock to acquiring accurate data. Older people state that they do not report crimes because: they do not believe police can recover stolen property, especially if it was not properly identified and marked; they believe reporting crime is a waste of the victim's and law enforcement officials' time; and they do not want to admit they have been victimized, thinking the admission may be viewed as a failure on their part.

This failure to report makes it difficult to determine the level of victimization, the only measure being the number of crimes reported to police. Yet, in the majority of police departments, the victim's age is not recorded in the report, thus adding to the inaccessibility of data on older people. Therefore, the FBI's Uniform Crime Report compiled from these data is a useless index of crime against the elderly.

Because many law enforcement officials are not aware of the special needs of elderly persons, changes in their attitudes toward, and responses to, elderly crime victims have been slow. The fact that most departments are not concerned about the age of their victims is an indication of their lack of knowledge about older persons' special needs. Law enforcement must foster the development of awareness among its officers—an awareness that the elderly victim requires a special response which embodies concern and compassion. Poor inner-city elderly residents are the most frequent non-reporters of crime (U.S., Congress, House, April 1977; Pope and Feyerherm, 1976). Unlike more affluent, better educated, middle-class older Americans, the poor inner-city elderly need direction. If police are considerate and attentive to elderly victims they will be encouraged to report future victimizations, thus contributing to accurate data.

With the advent of crime and the elderly as a "hot" issue, the statistical data generated by social scientists have proliferated haphazardly, promoting greater confusion. All statistical data can be interpreted in a number of ways, depending on the researcher and the situation. A prime example of this is a series of victimization surveys conducted for the Law Enforcement Assistance Administration (LEAA).

The LEAA's survey method, unlike the FBI's Uniform Crime Reports, does not rely on incidents reported to the police. The LEAA surveys have two main elements: a continuous national survey, and periodic surveys of selected central city areas. These surveys reveal that only one-third of crimes against older people are reported to police.

Five of the LEAA's city surveys constitute the most extensive documentation of victimization by different groups in our society. The surveys measure crimes considered most serious by the general public and crimes lending themselves to measurement by the survey method. Rape, robbery, assault, and personal larceny are the crimes against individuals measured by these surveys. Burglary, larceny, and motor vehicle theft are the crimes against households measured.

The Scope of the Problem

The surveys found that older persons are victims of violent crime at a rate of 8 per 1000 population, compared to a rate of 32 per 1000 for the general population. The rate for theft among the elderly is 22 per 1000 compared to 91 per 1000 for the general population; for household crimes, it is 107 per 1000 households, while for the general population it is 217 per 1000.

But other data reveal a different story. For example, "Criminal Victimization Surveys in the Nation's Five Largest Cities" (U.S., Congress, House, April 1977), shows that the elderly have the highest victimization rate for larceny involving bodily contact in four of the five cities surveyed.

The study, "Crime in Eight American Cities," documents a victimization rate for the general population for personal larceny with bodily contact of 317 per 100,000 population, compared to 342 per 100,000 for those aged 56–64 and 362 per 100,000 for persons 65 years and over. Robbery resulting in injury was highest for persons 50 years and above in three of the eight cities with the single exception of persons under 20 years of age.

According to LEAA's national survey figures for 1973 and 1974, the increase in crimes of violence against persons over 65 was second only to the increase against 16- to 19-year-old males. Assault against older people increased 46% during this one-year period. Personal larceny involving bodily contact also increased 14.4% for men. Robbery against males decreased 28.4% without injury, but rose 25.4% with injury.

Crimes of violence against both sexes increased 6.5% between 1973 and 1974 for those 65 and older, while theft against women 65 and older increased 11.7%, a larger increase than for any other age group. Personal larceny without bodily contact also increased 11.2% for women.

Household crimes against the elderly also increased dramatically during the 1973–74 period. Persons 65 and older had an increase in more kinds of household crimes (burglary, household larceny, and motor vehicle theft) than any other population group except the small number of households headed by persons under age 20.

A major drawback of these LEAA surveys is their failure to include certain crimes to which the elderly are more susceptible by virtue of their age, health, and economic status (Goldsmith and Tomas, 1974). Among these are fraud, confidence games, medical quackery, and harassment by teenagers. Many researchers of elderly crime victimization have failed to ensure that their data are complete and valid. Due to the "bandwagon" approach, most elderly victimization data cannot be used as the bases for generalizations concerning the aged and crime.

While we may not be able to accurately measure the extent of elderly crime victimization, we can draw the conclusion that the elderly are victims of certain types of crimes out of proportion to their number in the general population. This assumption is confirmed by studies in several cities.

According to a survey conducted in New York City in 1974, 15% of homicide victims were women over 65. This was greatly out of proportion to their percentage in the city's population. Another New York study found that 35% of the city's elderly lived in the twenty-six poorest neighborhoods; 40% of those interviewed reported being victimized. Similar problems were found in Oakland, California where women over 65 were victimized by robbers at the rate of one in twenty-four, compared to one in one hundred forty-six for those under 65. In Wilmington, Delaware, persons over 60, comprising only 19.7% of the city's population, were victims of twice as many street crimes as those under 60. A Boston, Massachusetts study reveals that the elderly made up 12% of the city's population, yet accounted for 28% of all robberies.

The California State Attorney General reported that in 1975 more than 90% of fraud and confidence game victims in Los Angeles and San Francisco were over 65 and were mostly women. The California medical quackery business takes in more than $50 million annually, and 70% of the reported cases involve elderly victims.

A study of the Houston Model Neighborhood Area (HMNA) in Texas, conducted between June 1971 and June 1973, revealed that for certain crimes such as robbery, swindling, purse snatching, and homicide, those 65 and over were more often victimized than those under 65 (Forston and Kitchens, 1974).

A Kansas City, Missouri study, "Patterns of Crimes Against Older

Americans," looked at serious crimes against persons 60 and older from Sept. 1, 1972–Apr. 15, 1975. During that time, 2,958 cases of burglary, robbery, purse snatching, assault, fraud, rape, and homicide occurred. Approximately 1,400 of these crimes were studied in detail. The rate of robbery was higher for the elderly than for any other group. In non-inner-city areas, the elderly were robbed at a rate approximately twice that of younger persons living in the same area. The inner-city elderly were robbed approximately four times more often than other age groups outside inner-city areas (Tighe, 1977).

Crimes that Plague the Elderly

The Subcommittee on Housing and Consumer Interests of the U.S. House Select Committee on Aging conducted a survey of chiefs of police in fifty cities around the country. Of the thirty-four who responded, ten reported that the elderly had higher victimization rates for certain crimes than other population groups. Atlanta reported higher rates in pedestrian robbery and swindling, Detroit, higher rates in unarmed robbery and breaking and entering, and Denver and Philadelphia, higher rates for robbery. Hartford, Conn. had higher rates for purse snatchings, muggings, and swindling. Higher rates for the elderly were reported in other cities as follows: Montgomery, Ala., con game artists and robbery; Montpelier, Vt., commerical fraud, medical quackery, insurance fraud, and high pressure sales schemes; San Antonio, Tex., con games and swindles; and Seattle, Wash., purse snatchings and crimes against the person. . . .

Examining the profiles of elderly victims obtained from these independent city surveys gives further insight into the impact. Poor inner-city elderly suffer from crime more often than their non-inner-city counterparts.

In Wilmington, Del., 86.7% of the victims surveyed were between the ages of 60 and 77; 72.6% were white women. The 105 persons surveyed had been victimized a total of 144 times after reaching age 60, and 41.4% had been injured. The crimes usually occurred within four blocks of their home, where 76% of the victims lived alone.

In Detroit, the average age of the victims was 67.8 years, and 12% were over age 80; 20% more women than men were victims. The majority were poor, with 68% having incomes under $3,500, and most of the remainder less than $7,000.

In Houston, 26% of all victims were elderly men and 32% women; 32% were black and 26%, white. Only 3% of the Houston sample had incomes above $10,000, 80% had incomes less than $5,000, and 16% had incomes between $5,000 and $10,000.

In Kansas City, blacks comprised 14.9% of the elderly population but accounted for 21.7% of the victimizations. This rate was almost 20% higher than the rate for whites. Elderly black men were victimized at a rate 75.4% higher than elderly white men, while the victimization rate for older black women was 39% higher than for white counterparts. Approximately 27.3% of the elderly were multiple victims. Blacks were multiple victims at a rate of slightly more than one in three, compared to whites who were multiple victims at a rate of one in four.

The Boston study revealed that criminals are more likely to use violence on older persons. Only 25.2% of victims under 60 years of age were injured (19.7% required hospital treatment), while 41.9% of the over-60 victims were injured and 27.5% needed hospital treatment.

Elderly vulnerability to crime is also increased by economic, physical, environmental, and social factors that are not fully examined in the cited studies. For example, the Bureau of Labor Statistics reported in 1973 that half of the aged couples in the United States had incomes below the amount ($5,414) that provided a "modest but adequate" standard of living. Thus, many elderly crime victims are poor both relatively and absolutely. A twenty dollar loss by theft for an elderly person with a fixed income is a much greater loss than the same amount stolen from an employed younger person. If robbed, most older persons have no reserve funds to use until the next social security or pension check arrives. If property is taken from an older person, the financial capability to replace it is less than for a younger person.

Many older persons also experience diminished physical strength and stamina. Statistics indicate more than 60% of the elderly live in metropolitan areas, and most of these reside in the central city. For cultural, emotional, and economic reasons, many elderly have lived in the same area for decades. Many cannot afford alternative housing, and they are often dependent on public transportation. These urban elderly are consequently close to those most likely to victimize them—the unemployed, drug addicts, and teenage school dropouts. Criminals often know when social security, SSI, and pension checks are delivered, and can therefore judge with accuracy when an older person will be carrying cash.

Older persons are also more likely to be multiple victims of the same crimes (Goldsmith, 1975). Additionally, the elderly cannot move away from their home area and, fearing reprisals, often do not report being victimized.

Fear of Crime

The psychological impact of fear of crime is another aspect of criminal victimization that the cited studies do not address. The 1974 Louis Harris and Associates national survey of the problems of the elderly found that they rank fear of crime as their most serious problem—above health, money, and loneliness. A 1971 Los Angeles *Times* poll found fear of crime second only to economics as a cause of stress among the elderly. In two studies sponsored by the National Retired Teachers Association/Association of Retired Persons in 1972 and 1973, more than 80,000 older persons were surveyed and indicated that fear of crime ranked second in their lives, following concern about adequate food and shelter.

The Louis Harris poll reported that persons with low incomes are more fearful of victimization than others. Of those with incomes under $3,000 per year, 31% felt fear of crime was a major social problem, while only 17% of those with incomes of $15,000 or more expressed that fear. This relationship between income and fear of crime may be explained by the fact that poorer people live more often in high-crime, inner-city neighborhoods and actually experience greater victimization than the wealthier suburban elderly.

Virtually all studies have found a higher fear of crime among elderly blacks than among elderly whites. The Harris survey of older people found 21% of the white population stated crime was a serious personal problem, while 41% of the blacks surveyed reported fear of crime. The survey also found a correlation between race and income and fear of crime. Of those with incomes less than $3,000, 28% of the whites and 44% of the blacks said that fear of crime was a very serious problem. For persons with incomes over $3600, these percentages dropped to 18% for whites and 33% for blacks.

Frank Clemente and Michael B. Kleiman (1976) found 47% of the elderly white population they studied feared walking alone in their neighborhoods, compared to 60% of the elderly blacks in their survey. A number of studies have examined the nature of elderly fear of victimization and how it is distributed. A study by the National Opinion Research Center at the University of Chicago revealed 34% of older men and 69% of elderly women reported fear of crime as a grave concern.

Community size appears to be related to the fear of crime victimization. According to Harris polls in 1964, 1966, 1967, 1969, and 1970, as well as Gallup polls in 1967, 1968, and 1972, the fear of victimization increases along with the size of the community in which older persons live. Clemente and Kleiman also found fear of victimization "decreases in a clear step pattern as one moves from large cities to rural areas."

Due to incomplete data, the extent of elderly victimization cannot be accurately measured. However, the studies we have cited do provide convincing evidence that a higher proportion of older Americans are victims of certain types of crimes than the general population. The testimony of older victims and local officials also supports the conclusion that the consequences of victimization are frequently more devastating (U.S., Congress, House, December 1976). This is especially true for fraud, as pointed out by Robert Butler in his book, *Why Survive? Being Old in America* (1975). He suggests there are several factors that contribute to the general vulnerability of older persons to fraud including loneliness, grief, chronic illness, lack of education, the desire to be young again, and low income levels.

The elderly are being victimized. We can and must work to alleviate this problem.

Editor's Comment

There is no evidence that young people are more prone than old to report crimes, to believe that police do recover stolen property, to admit that they have been victimized, nor are the police specially sensitive to needs of other groups. In addition, criminology is no more an exact discipline than are the other social sciences (Gertz and Talarico, 1977). Its statistics are even less accurate than those of other social disciplines. While this statement may not apply to LEAA survey data, crime statistics are almost infinitely malleable and the temptation to manipulate them for political ends is great. For example, a criminal act may be called rape (a felony) or carnal knowledge (a misdemeanor).

Arguments presented by Malinchak and Wright (1978) for greater vulnerability to crime of older people apply equally well to other low income groups; the young poor can equally little afford to lose their property to criminals who prey on inner-city dwellers or to have their welfare checks stolen.

Skipping around the country, they present evidence gained by a survey of chiefs of police in various cities, that elderly are more likely to be victimized by con men in Montgomery, Alabama, by unarmed robbery in Detroit, purse snatching in Hartford, and so on. Given the notorious inaccuracy of crime statistics in general, which the authors note selectively (that many researchers of *elderly* crime victimization have failed to ensure that their data are complete and valid), what is one to make of such selective data as they present? When the police budget comes up for review, crimes may be shifted to the felony end in order to show the need for more police; when the Chief makes his report to the city fathers, acts will more likely be defined as misdemeanors, to show the marvelous efficiency of the police.

Evaluating the Rhetoric of Crisis: A Case Study of Criminal Victimization of the Elderly*

F. Cook and T. Cook

Much biological and social evidence indicates that shifts in established forms of behavior often take place in response to perceived crises. As Marmor and Kudrle (1975) have suggested for the policy sciences, defining a problem as a crisis focuses attention on that issue and may help to organize action aimed at solving it. Therefore, there is often a rationale for making rhetorical allusions to crisis when seeking support for a particular course of political action. However, it is important for policy-makers not to get so caught up in the rhetoric of crisis that they fail to make a detailed analysis of the relationship between the nature of the problem specified in the rhetoric and the nature of the problem indicated by available data. Sometimes, the crisis rhetoric and the analysis of data will result in a common definition of the issue to be resolved. But at other times the two processes may lead to different definitions, and the problem implied by the rhetoric may be less serious than the one implied by the data. Since resources for tackling problems are usually limited, they are more usefully directed at empirically demonstrated problems rather than at those indicated by rhetoric.

This article examines a case in which the rhetoric of crisis has been used. Claims have been made that victimization of the elderly has reached "crisis" proportions. After documenting these claims, we propose four definitions of what might constitute a crisis of victimization. Data are then presented in order to test whether the crisis of rhetoric is appropriate according to any definition of a crisis.

*For space reasons, the six tables in the original report have been omitted. Interested readers should consult these tables for an understanding of how large or small are particular relationships involving the elderly. Also, though the data reported here do not go beyond 1973, national victimization survey data for 1974, 1975, and 1976 show similar relationships.

Public Statements: The Elderly and Their "Crisis" of Victimization

Since 1971, criminal victimization of the elderly seems to have captured more and more of the attention of scholars, members of the legislative and executive branches of government, and journalists. At the congressional level, many case studies describing crimes against the elderly in federally funded housing projects were presented to the 1971 Senate Subcommittee on Housing for the Elderly (U.S., Congress, Senate, October 1971). At the next year's hearings, Senator Harrison Williams went beyond the problem of the elderly in public housing by stating: "Elderly tenants in private and public housing in many of our big cities are the most vulnerable victims of theft, violence, rowdyism, and outright terrorism . . . Many older persons lock themselves within their apartments night and day and dread every knock on the door. Do we need any more proof that a crisis in crime exists? Do we need any more reason to act on an emergency basis?" (U.S., Congress, Senate, August 1972). Senator Kennedy went even farther at a hearing two months later and stated: "The threat of crime and violence against our older citizens demands a response from all levels of government. . . . A decent and safe living environment is an inherent right of all elderly citizens." (U.S., Congress, Senate, October 1972). Senators Williams and Kennedy have not been alone in drawing attention to the problem, as is attested by the remarks of Senator Ribicoff in the Congressional Record of September 24, 1975, or the remarks of Senator Beall in the same source for the next day.

The executive branch's interest in criminal victimization of the elderly may have been heightened by the 1973 White House Conference on Aging at which the recommendation was made that "police protection of the elderly should become a top priority" (White House Conference on Aging, 1973). President Ford explicitly mentioned crimes against the elderly in his September 5, 1975, speech before the California legislature as well as in his June 1975 message on crime to Congress when he said: "Most of the victims of violent crimes are the poor, the old, the young, the disadvantaged minorities" (Ford, 1975). And Arthur S. Flemming, President Ford's Commissioner of Aging, spoke at the 1975 National Conference on Crimes against the Elderly in order to urge collaboration among federal agencies to create "a meaningful pool of resources to deal with crime against older Americans" (Flemming, 1975).

At least three different scholars have drawn attention to the frequency of crimes against the elderly. First, Carl Cunningham of the Midwest Research Institute spoke about his research at the 1975 Conference on

Crimes against the Elderly, and his conclusion was widely reported nationally: that "the elderly living in or near certain neighborhoods of Kansas City, Missouri, can be as much as eight times more vulnerable to serious crimes . . . than a young resident of a relatively safe suburb" (Cunningham, 1975). Next, Goldsmith and Tomas published an article on "Crimes against the Elderly: A Continuing National Crisis" in the journal *Aging*, a publication of the Administration on Aging distributed among various public and private groups active in the aging policy arena. The article concluded that "the elderly constitute a unique class of crime victims and . . . crimes against the elderly can be considered a distinct category of criminal activity" (Goldsmith and Tomas, 1974; Goldsmith and Goldsmith, 1975). Finally, Robert Butler, head of the National Institute on Aging, devoted a chapter in his book *Why Survive? Being Old in America* to "Victimization of the Elderly," and, without citing relevant evidence, he stated: "Old people are victims of violent crime more than any other age group" (Butler, 1975).

It should not be thought that the evidence we have just cited is buried in unread reports or books. Most of it was reported in the national press, including excerpts from the testimony at Senator Williams's subcommittee meetings, President Ford's addresses to both Congress and the California legislature, and the research findings of both Cunningham, and Goldsmith and Tomas. These are not, however, the only media references to the special victimization plight of the elderly. For instance, the CBS evening news of February 28, 1976 carried a story about crimes against the elderly in Delaware and cited a study which claimed to show that purse snatchings were twice as frequent in that city against persons over sixty than against younger persons (Rather, 1976).

It would probably be wrong to maintain that criminal victimization of the elderly is currently very high on the agenda of the groups responsible for dealing with the problems of the elderly or victims of crime. Rather, it would be more judicious to conclude that the public statements we have just cited could result in elevating the national profile of the problem. This consequence would presumably be all the more likely if the "rhetoric of crisis" were widely held to be appropriate for describing the plight of the elderly.

Is There a National Crisis of Victimization of the Elderly?

To test whether the language of crisis is appropriate for describing the current state of victimization of the elderly, we need to define *crisis*. It is not easy to define the term in a way that would suit all persons. However, we think that four types of evidence need to be examined to establish whether it is warranted to label a given state of empirical affairs a "crisis" of victimization. One type of evidence concerns the *relative frequency* of victimization, and the issue here is: Are the elderly more likely than other subgroups of the population to be victimized?

A second type of evidence relates to *increases in the rate of victimization*. The issue here is: Is victimization increasing at a faster rate for the elderly than for other groups?

A third type of evidence concerns the *relative severity of consequences*. The issues here are: Are the elderly more likely than others to suffer from violent crimes, and for any given type of crime, are the elderly likely to be hurt more by its consequences? For example, are they robbed of more money than other groups, or if they are robbed of similar amounts, is the loss greater in proportion to what they have to lose?

The final type of evidence relates to the *relative fear of being victimized*. The issue is: Are the elderly more fearful than others of being victims, regardless of whether their fears are in accord with statistical evidence about the probability and consequences of their being victimized?

Data from a variety of sources exist for answering the first, second, and fourth questions. This article will examine the relevant evidence. Usually, more than one set of data will be reported for answering each question, thereby permitting an assessment of the replicability of findings. Unfortunately, no data are presently available for answering some subparts of the third question concerning the relative severity of the consequences of senior citizen victimization. In particular, one cannot answer whether the elderly suffer more from crimes of comparable severity, though we can answer whether they are disproportionately overvictimized when it comes to the more severe categories of crime, especially violent crimes.

Frequency of victimization. The best social science data on the frequency of victimization in the United States inevitably come from national surveys on representative samples. Two such surveys can be examined. The earlier one was conducted by the National Opinion Research Center (NORC) in 1966 and involved a full-scale multistage probability sample of 10,000 households in the continental United States (Ennis, 1967). The study was designated to measure the amount of criminal victimization in the United States by asking people which crimes had been committed against them during the preceding year. The data [show] that in the adult age categories, the elderly (defined as 60 and over) are least likely to be the victims of most classes of crime.

In 1973 a survey was authorized by the Law Enforcement Assistance

Administration (LEAA) of the U.S. Department of Justice and was conducted by the U.S. Bureau of the Census (U.S., Department of Justice,
LEAA, 1975). Its purpose was to gauge the extent to which persons age 12
and over, households, and businesses report having been criminally victimized during a twelve-month period. The sample was a probability
sample consisting of 60,000 households in the fifty states and the District of
Columbia. Within each household, questions were asked of all individual
household members who were 12 and over. Crimes were categorized as
those against persons (rape, robbery, assault, and personal larceny) and
those against households (burglary, household larceny, and motor vehicle
theft).

The LEAA survey treated age in a slightly different fashion from the
NORC survey and defined the aged as 65 and over rather than 60 and over.
Nevertheless, once again the data show that older persons are the least
likely age group to be the victims of most personal crimes. On the whole,
about 32 elderly persons per 1000 were victims of personal crimes, whereas the rate was 201 per 1000 for persons age 20 to 24 and about 136 per 1000
for persons aged 25 to 34. Moreover, the overall rate tends to decrease with
age. The same pattern holds true for crimes against households. Among the
elderly, about 109 per 1000 were victims as opposed to 302 per 1000 for 20
to 34 year olds and 251 per 1000 for 35 to 49 year olds.

Could there be alternative interpretations of the age effect in the
NORC and LEAA data? Five such interpretations might be raised. First,
the effect may be due to the reduced number of crime categories that apply
to the elderly. For example, we would expect the elderly to be less subject
to motor vehicle theft since fewer old people drive, and we would expect
elderly women to be less subject to rape because sexual attraction plays
some role in the selection of victims and most elderly women would be less
attractive to younger rapists. However, this possible explanation of the age
effect is not likely, for negative correlations between age and victimization
persist across all crime classifications discussed above, except perhaps for
robbery without injury, where the 65 and older group is victimized more
than their slightly younger cohorts but not more than most other age
groups. Thus, the relative immunity of the aged to victimization is not
restricted to a few categories of crime.

A second possible interpretation is that the effects of age cannot be
distinguished from the effects of sex. That is, if males are victimized more
than females and males die earlier than females, then the lower victimization rate for all persons over 65 could simply reflect the fact that there are
fewer aged males than females. However, a separate breakdown of the
victimization data by sex reveals that victimization decreases significantly
with age for both males and females (U.S., Department of Justice, LEAA,

1975). Thus, sex differences in mortality cannot account for age differences in victimization.

A third possibility is that the age effect is due to age being confounded with race. That is, the lesser victimization of the aged might simply be because whites are victimized less than blacks and whites constitute a higher percentage of the aged than of the young. Though the reports we previously considered did not break down the data by both race and age, a 1973 survey did. The results of the analysis show that a negative correlation between age and victimization holds for both blacks and whites, thereby ruling out the possibility that the global relationship of age and victimization is due to a confounding of age and race.

A fourth explanation might be that the relationship of age and victimization rate is limited to comparisons of senior citizens with teenagers and very young adults and that there is no general correlation between the two. Though the data indicate that crimes against persons are most heavy among the age group 12 to 24 (with less violent crimes from 12 to 15 and more violent ones from 16 to 24), there is nonetheless a negative relationship all across the age distribution. Hence, victimization tends to be less the older one is, even when the 35 to 64 age range is considered apart from the youngest and oldest.

A final speculation is that the age differences in victimization may be due to reporting biases. For instance, it may be that elderly people have worse memories and so report a lower percentage of the victimizations they actually experienced than do younger persons. However, though the biological basis of memory does deteriorate with age, memory is not the only determinant of recall, and it does not seem plausible to us that elderly persons contemplate less than younger persons such experiences as robbery or larceny. Indeed, the opposite may be true. We can think of no age-related reporting biases that would be large enough to account for all or most of the observed relationship between age and victimization.

To conclude, while we cannot assess the cumulative effect of these five potential sources of bias, none of them can singly account for the fact that reported victimization tends to decrease with age. Indeed, the relationship can be observed across a variety of racial, sex, and age groups and across a variety of crimes.

Increase in the rate of victimization. The NORC and LEAA samples are not entirely comparable, and great caution must be exercised in using the studies to estimate how victimization rates changed between 1966 and 1973. However, gross comparisons are possible by examining the NORC data for 1966 and the LEAA data for 1973 in impressionistic fashion.

As far as the aged are concerned, for those measures that are common to each survey, there appears to be no dramatic increase over time in the probability of being victimized. For aggravated assaults in 1966, the rate was 1.5 per 1000 when persons 60 and over were the victims and in 1973 the rate was 1.2 per 1,000 for persons 65 and over. (It is not possible to compute these rates on the same age basis without making tenuous assumptions.) Compare these rates with those for younger victims: 3.39 for persons 10 to 19 in 1966 and about 20.0 for persons 12 to 19 in 1973. With respect to robbery, persons 60 and over in 1966 had a rate of about one per 1,000, while in 1973 persons 65 and over had a rate of 4.8 per 1,000 when robberies with and without injuries are considered. Compare these estimates with those for persons age 10 to 19 in 1973: 0.6 per 1,000; and age 12 to 19 in 1973: about 11 per 1,000. In all cases, victimization of the elderly appears to be increasing over time in an absolute sense, but there is no indication that it is growing at a faster rate than for other age groups. Indeed, the trends are all in the opposite direction, though it must be acknowledged that differences in definitions among surveys make it impossible to be definitive. All we can conclude is that the evidence does not suggest that victimization of the elderly is increasing at a faster rate than the victimization of other age groups.

Severity of the consequences of being victimized. The rhetoric of "crisis" would be partly justified if it could be established that elderly persons suffer more than younger persons when they are victimized. One way in which they might suffer more would be if they were disproportionately subjected to crimes involving violence. But this is not the case. In 1966 the elderly were least likely to be the victims of aggravated assault, while in 1973 the elderly were least likely to be the victims of aggravated assault, simple assault, and robbery with injury.

A second way in which the elderly might suffer more severe consequences would be if, despite the lower incidence of being victims, the physical and economic consequences of a given type of victimization were more for them than for others. This could happen, for example, because the elderly are frailer and so feel more pain or need longer periods in the hospital to recover, or because they are poorer and so the loss of even small sums of money dramatically affects their disposable income. There are not yet data available, however, which relate age to the severity of the physical or economic consequences of being victimized. Until then, only anecdotal evidence exists about the special economic, social, and medical vulnerability of the aged. Much of this evidence stresses how much the elderly suffer when they are victimized, and it is not difficult to make readers feel anguish at the description of an aged woman who is savagely attacked and robbed of her life savings. While we know that such events occur relatively less frequently than with other age groups, we do not yet know whether the dramatic cases portrayed in the media are representative of how much the elderly suffer physically or economically when they are victimized in the same way that younger persons are.

Fear of being victimized. Past experience with crime, or anticipation of future crime, can have psychological effects, so we need to know whether older Americans are more fearful than others of being victimized or of suffering negative consequences should they be victimized. Fortunately, data exist on the public's fear of crime. The National Opinion Research Center is currently studying changes in social attitudes since 1948 among four age cohorts (Adams and Smith, forthcoming): a new cohort (those born after 1940), a young cohort (those born from 1925 to 1940), a middle cohort (born from 1910 to 1925), and an old cohort (born before 1910). The cohorts' fear of crime was measured in 1965, 1967, and 1968 by the American Institute of Public Opinion (AIPO, or Gallup Poll) and in 1973 and 1974 by the NORC General Social Surveys. In all five surveys, fear of crime was determined by respondents' answers to the question, "Is there any area right around here—that is, within a mile— where you would be afraid to walk alone at night?" This question does not specifically address the problem of fear of crime. Rather, it probes the respondents' fear of walking in their neighborhoods. However, it can reasonably be assumed that if a person is afraid of walking in his neighborhood, he is afraid of crime there.

The data indicate that the oldest cohort was most fearful in each of the five years the surveys were conducted. About 38% of the elderly expressed fear in 1965, 33% in 1967, 41% in 1968, 46% in 1973, and 56% in 1974. The percentages for the youngest group were lower: 35, 30, 37, 40, and 43%, respectively. What is most important, though, is that the difference between the oldest and youngest cohorts seems to have dramatically increased. In 1965 the difference was about 3%, in 1967 it was still 3%, in 1968 it was 4%, in 1973 it was 6%, and in 1974 it was 14%. Thus, fear of crime appears to have increased at a faster rate among the elderly than among the young.

Does this fear cause the elderly to stay home more than other subgroups of the population? If so, are the elderly least likely to be victimized because they are least likely to be available for attack on the streets and most likely to be at home to avoid robbery? A recent study conducted for the National Council on the Aging by Louis Harris and Associates found that people 65 and over visit movies, sporting events, public parks, libraries, live artistic performances, museums, and restaurants less often than persons aged 18 to 64 and that it is only for visiting churches or synagogues that the elderly go out more than the young (by 3%) (Harris, 1975). However, the fact that most of the elderly go out less often does not by itself "prove" that they stay home because of a fear of crime. Since the respondents in the study were not asked why they stayed home, the reader is left wondering whether income, accessibility, mobility, fear, or some other factor provides the answer. The reader is also left wondering whether the degree to which the elderly go out accounts for their lower chances of being victimized either on the street or in the home.

One way to answer this would be to use leisure surveys to learn how much time various age groups spend on the street or out of the home and then to use these estimates to compute the ratio of the victimization rate both to the time spent on the street and to the time spent out of the home. Though we do not want to prejudge the results of such an analysis, it may not entirely eliminate the relationship between age and victimization rate. This is because the relationship holds across a variety of age groups between 30 and 65, and these groups may not differ appreciably either in time spent out of the home or in time spent on the street.

Which age group is most victimized?   The young are the most likely age group to be victimized. In 1973, about 236 per 1000 of the 12 to 15 year olds and 237 per 1000 of the 16 to 19 year olds were victims of crimes against persons, as compared with about 32 per 1000 of those over 65. Other data from LEAA show that income is negatively related to being the victim of crimes of violence but is positively related to being the victim of crimes without violence. Thus, families with incomes of less than $3,000 are most likely to have had robberies or assaults perpetrated on their members, while families with incomes over $15,000 are most likely to have been victims of larceny (U.S., Department of Justice, LEAA, 1975).

The LEAA and NORC data also show that blacks are more heavily victimized than whites in crimes of violence (rape, robbery, and assault); moreover, poor blacks are more likely to suffer robbery and assault than more affluent blacks. Thus, the profile of the most typical victim of robbery and assault is a young, black, and poor male.

Other data also indicate that the young are increasingly being victimized. The Senate Subcommittee to Investigate Juvenile Delinquency conducted a mail questionnaire survey of 757 public school districts throughout the United States with an enrollment of 10,000 pupils or more (U.S., Congress, Senate, Committee on the Judiciary, 1975). The response rate was high, 68.1% (516 school districts). Though the subcommittee's report did not deal with other age groups and so no comparative baseline is available, there are nonetheless increases in the rate with which students were victimized. For instance, between 1970 and 1973: (1) homicides increased by 18.5%; (2) rapes and attempted rapes increased by 40.1%; (3) robberies increased by 36.7%; (4) assaults on students increased by 85.3%; (5) assaults on teachers increased by 77.4%; (6) burglaries of school buildings increased by 11.8%; (7) drug and alcohol offenses on school property increased by 37.5%; (8) dropouts increased by 11.7%; and (9) weapons confiscated by school authorities rose by 54.4%.

Implications of the Findings

It is difficult to discuss victimization of the elderly in a comprehensive context since we do not yet know if the elderly suffer more than others when they are victimized. However, the data presently available suggest that the major policy problem associated with the elderly and crime is probably not crime per se. Rather, the problem is related to the elderly person's fear of crime and the restrictions to daily mobility that this fear may impose. If it is the case that the currently available data do not support the "crisis" labelling, what were the bases for past claims that the victimization of the elderly had reached crisis proportions? Most of the claims were based on heart-rending individual case studies of elderly victims which, while dramatic, gave no clues either to the absolute frequency of victimization of aged persons or to their victimization rate relative to younger persons. Other claims were based on inappropriate age comparisons, as when elderly persons in high-crime areas were compared with younger persons in low-crime areas rather than with the young in their own neighborhoods. But it should be firmly borne in mind that only the NORC 1966 data were available when the crisis rhetoric began. Hence, persons using such language cannot be blamed for failing to consider systematic data, most of which did not exist in published form when they made their claims.

If the "fear diagnosis" in this article is correct, it suggests that the policy response to victimization of the elderly should be targeted at alleviating fear. This response might well include campaigns to inform older persons that they are not being singled out as victims and that talk of a crisis of victimization is unwarranted unless it is understood to mean a fear of victimization. It should also be noted that a fear diagnosis might require less capital-intensive programs than would a "victimization diagnosis," for the latter could entail human or canine patrols and expensive technological devices.

Four limitations to our fear diagnosis need mentioning. First, the fear data are based on a single questionnaire item, albeit an item that was asked in five separate years. Second, we do not yet know whether the physical and economic consequences of being victimized are more serious for the elderly even though they, as a group, are victimized less often than other groups. Third, we do not yet know whether elderly persons would continue to be victimized less than younger persons after one has taken account of the fact that elderly people probably spend less time out of doors. It is important to know this, for if fear were reduced and the elderly spent more time outside and became victimized even more because of this, then alleviating their fear might do more harm than good. Fourth, we define "crisis" in relative rather than absolute terms; even though crimes against the elderly are increasing and each one may arouse a special moral indignation, we nonetheless persist in defining the victimization problem of the elderly relative to that of other age groups.

Why is it useful or necessary to define criminal victimization of the elderly in relative rather than absolute terms? It is a fact of policy life that a variety of social problems compete for a finite quantity of attention and funds. Claims that victimization of the elderly has reached crisis proportions may serve to mobilize public attention and support behind the elderly. But at whose cost? Our fear is that, if the plight of elderly crime victims becomes even more visible nationally, more resources will be devoted to them at the cost of poor, young, black males, who are in fact the most likely victims (and perpetrators) of crime in the United States today. Reassessing priorities and shifting attention to the elderly does not necessarily make the victimization problems that were formerly top priority go away—and the problem of poor, black males has not gone away. Just as it can be dangerous to shift agendas when the items of the old agenda were not solved, so it can be dangerous to redefine priorities when persisting problems have not been solved. We should consider in detail whether the very real plight of the elderly who are victimized deserves to be labeled a crisis, and whether our genuine sympathy for them should stand in the way of determining priorities by data-based criteria rather than by short-term political considerations or by a genuine and spontaneous concern for a relatively small number of elderly persons.

Editor's Comment

The authors of both papers were afforded an opportunity to present rebuttals. Malinchak's rebuttal arrived too late to be used. The Cooks did reply as follows.

Criminal Victimization of the Elderly:
Is the Crisis Rhetoric Warranted Yet?

F. Cook and T. Cook

We shall discuss four of the major substantive issues raised by Malinchak and Wright:

1. For certain crimes victimization rates are higher for the elderly than for other age groups.

2. The rate of increase in crime is greater for the elderly than for the non-elderly.

3. The consequences of being victimized are greater for the elderly than for other age groups.

4. Elderly persons in inner city areas are victimized at a higher rate than are younger persons.

Crime Rates

First, Malinchak and Wright use *data from a variety of cities* to claim that for certain crimes victimization rates are higher for the elderly than for other age groups. In our article, we saw how the NORC and LEAA survey data suggested that *nationwide* victimization rates are lower for the elderly for all household crimes (burglary, larceny, and auto theft) and for most personal crimes (rape, robbery, with injury, aggravated assault, simple assault, and personal larceny). The only exception was for robbery without injury where adults over 65 were victimized more than adults 34 and older but less than persons under 35. Closer analysis of the LEAA data (Cook et al., 1978) has shown that these robberies without injury are mostly purse-snatchings (the larcenies with body contact mentioned by Malinchak and Wright) and that the elderly are victimized more often in this category when compared to adults over 34, but considerably less than persons between 12 and 34. The major differences between Malinchak and Wright and us on this particular substantive issue are trivial. The conclusions are basically in agreement, and only the interpretations different. They stress the one crime category where the elderly are victimized more than other adults over 34; we see this one category in a broader context of many other crimes, all of which show lower victimization rates for the elderly.

Malinchak and Wright correctly note that it is important to learn how age is related to special types of crime that could particularly affect the elderly, especially "fraud, confidence games, medical quackery, and harassment by teenagers." Two points need to be made about their suggestion. First, data about such crimes are included in the LEAA surveys as part of the more global crime categories like larceny without contact or robbery. However, such crimes are not so disproportionately targeted against the elderly that, within the crime category as a whole, the elderly are more frequent victims than younger persons. Second, something is known about harassment by teenagers, at least when a crime is committed. National survey data have shown (Antunes et al., 1977) that *when the elderly are victimized* they are more likely than others to be approached by young persons (rather than older criminals) acting alone (rather than in gangs) who are black (rather than white), who do not carry weapons, and who are not personally known to the elderly victim. This is not the picture of greater harassment of the elderly by gangs of teenagers. Instead, the picture is that when the elderly are victimized, it is by unknown young, inexperienced criminals acting alone.

Malinchak and Wright buttress their case for higher victimization rates on *selected* statistics for *selected* crimes in *selected* cities. The reader has no sense either (a) of the quality of studies in question, or (b) of the extent to which Malinchak and Wright's reporting capitalized on chance deviations (see Cook and Campbell, 1979, pp. 42–43); and (c) of the extent to which their findings, if valid, are generalizable. Take, for example, the first study mentioned in the list of city studies. It suggested that 15% of the murders in New York were of elderly persons, a higher percentage than the elderly constitute in that city's population. Contrast this with nationwide Uniform Crime Report (UCR) data on murder, a crime for which there is little underreporting. The UCR data for murder in 1973 (reported in Cook et al., 1978) show that 6% of the national murders of persons 12 and older involved victims over 65; yet persons over 65 constituted slightly more than 10% of the population.

Another example of the interpretative problems with Malinchak and Wright's reporting is their comparison of crime rates for black and white elderly, showing that the black elderly are victimized at higher rates. While an important descriptive finding, this is irrelevant to the issue addressed in our article and in much of Malinchak and Wright's paper, where the concern is with whether victimization rates increase with age among blacks and whites and with whether the rate of age-linked change in victimization rates is steeper for blacks than whites. With respect to these issues, we know from 1973 national data reported in our article that nearly all crimes decreased with age among both blacks and whites and that the rates of decrease do not seem to be different. Thus, though the black elderly are victimized more than white elderly, this is merely part of a trend for all blacks to be victimized more than whites at all ages.

Rate of Increase

A second difference between Malinchak and Wright and ourselves is with respect to the rate of increase in crimes against the elderly. Using non-comparable data sets spanning a seven year period we tentatively suggested that crime was increasing among all age groups but not at a faster rate among the elderly. Malinchak and Wright use LEAA national data for 1973 and 1974 to argue that in this one year period crimes of violence and household crimes increased at a faster rate against the elderly (men and women combined) than for any other age group other than youths. To show that these figures are likely to involve the biased selection of unstable estimates that lead to some large chance differences, we used published LEAA data for 1973 and 1976 to look at these same variables over a four year lag. Doing this showed that (a) crimes of violence decreased among the elderly and at a faster rate than for all other groups—the opposite conclusion to what Malinchak and Wright reported!; (b) the total assaults against elderly people, which increased by 46% between 1973 and 1974, stayed constant between 1973 and 1976, whereas they increase for most other mature adults; and (c) that household larcenies did indeed increase at a faster rate against homes where the head of the family was over 65, but burglaries against such homes *decrease at a faster rate!* By capitalizing upon chance fluctuations between two years and failing to examine the longer range picture, Malinchak and Wright have inadvertently given a false impression of how crimes are increasing against the elderly relative to other age groups. This set of errors was also made in the report *In Search of Security: A National Perspective* (U.S., Congress, House, April 1977) from which Malinchak and Wright derived their data about changes in victimization rates.

Consequences of Victimization

The third apparent difference between the two articles concerns the consequences of being victimized. Malinchak and Wright assert that the elderly suffer more from economic crimes because the loss of a given sum of money means more when one has a lower income. A related point often made, though not by Malinchak and Wright, is that the elderly, being frailer, also suffer more physically when violence is used. We, on the other hand, were cautious in our article suggesting, first, that little is known about age-related consequences of victimization and, second, that these consequences might not be especially serious for the elderly since the elderly were less likely to be the victims of more serious crimes. Since our article, we have published a paper on the age-linked consequences of crime (Cook et al., 1978), in which we used national survey data from LEAA. We showed that the elderly lost less than others in absolute dollar terms, were no more likely to suffer catastrophic losses (defined as a loss exceeding one month's income), but that they lost slightly more than other mature adults—i.e. persons over 34—when the amount lost is divided by income. We also showed that elderly victims were no more likely than others to need medical care, to receive medical care at some expense, or to receive more expensive medical treatment. When victimized, therefore, the elderly do not seem to suffer more than others in terms of the total amount of money lost or the injuries caused, and this may be because the modal crime against them is purse-snatching by inexperienced and un-armed youths acting alone. However, the financial loss relative to income is higher for persons over 65 than for persons between 27 and 64, though it is less than for persons under 27. Whether the elderly suffer more *from identical crimes* is an important issue to which we do not yet have any responsible answer.

Inner City Poor Elderly

Malinchak and Wright report from some city surveys that the elderly in inner city areas are victimized at a higher rate than younger persons and that this difference is greater than found in non-inner city areas. It seems, then, that it is the elderly trapped in inner city areas who disproportionate-ly suffer from crime. We have no national representative data comparing inner city areas to others. But we do have national representative data relating victimization to both age and total family income. On the assump-tion that inner city persons are more likely than others to be poor, we can very indirectly test Malinchak and Wright's assertion by seeing if elderly poor persons are victimized more than non-elderly poor persons and by testing whether this difference is larger than for more affluent elderly and non-elderly persons. We used the 1977 LEAA national data to do the appropriate analysis and found the opposite. That is, elderly and non-elderly persons with higher family incomes had more similar victimization profiles than elderly and non-elderly persons with lower family incomes! Moreover, among persons with lower incomes it was the young rather than the old who were victimized more. The implication of this is that we should be cautious in believing whether the poor elderly are victimized especially often. While victimization rates may in general be higher for the poor than the non-poor elderly, they are still less for the poor elderly than for non-elderly. Indeed, the difference between the more affluent elderly and non-elderly may be much less than the difference between the less affluent elderly and non-elderly.

What can be stated with confidence about crime and the elderly? At this time, it seems to us warranted to believe that: (a) the elderly are victimized less than others in nearly all crime categories; (b) when victimized, the elderly suffer offenses that are less serious in nature—the modal crime against the elderly seems to be purse-snatchings by inexperienced black youths acting alone; (c) the offenses perpetrated against the elderly do not cause any more physical harm than the offenses committed against younger persons; (d) the dollar losses caused by personal and household crimes are no greater for the elderly than others, but the loss relative to income is greater for the elderly than for other adults provided they are 27 or older; (e) the elderly fear crime more than others; but (f) they are no more likely than others to report changing their behavior because of a fear of crime (Cook et al., forthcoming). This picture differs from that of Malinchak and Wright. We suspect they have inadvertently chosen their evidence in a way that supports a case rather than letting the better quality data suggest how high a profile crime against the elderly should receive when compared to crime against other age groups. The losers in nearly all our analyses have been young persons under about 27.

Part Six

A Potpourri of Issues

12

Fashions, Faddism, and Quackery in Aging

It is better to know nothing than to know what ain't so.
Old New England Proverb.

In earlier chapters, many erroneous, irrational, and merely silly ideas about aging have been presented. There are many odds and ends of such foibles that do not warrant overexposure, yet should be briefly mentioned, so that those interested can further investigate these issues on their own.

Unbalanced Stereotypes of Aging

The introduction to this volume noted that while many texts and other volumes are exceedingly optimistic about biological and medical advances in aging (about which there can be much doubt), they are almost uniformly pessimistic about social conditions of the aging and discuss the aged as a "social problem." Ignored are the realities that the aged are a heterogenous group. As Binstock (1978) noted earlier, aged differ in race, sex, socioeconomic status, health, and every other variable, including age. There are few common features in the lives and attitudes of an early-retired 60-year-old, upper-level civil servant and an 80-year-old retired factory laborer.

A Harris Survey study (1975) is a gold mine of iconoclasm about the aged. It is a volume worth more than a casual leafing-through by any serious student of gerontology. Some examples:

Television viewing: A 68% majority believes that most older persons spend their time "watching TV a lot." Yet only 36% of those 65 and older said they watch TV frequently, compared with 23% of those under 65 who do so.

Inactivity: A substantial 66% of the 1,473 persons under 65 surveyed said they think that older persons just "sit around and think a lot," and assume that they have nothing better to do. Yet only 31% of those 65 and over say they do, compared with 37% of those under 65 who indicate that they sit around and think often. The survey also discovered that younger persons grossly underestimate the amount of activity that older persons engage in.

Loneliness: A 61% majority of the younger group believes that loneliness was a "very serious problem" for the elderly. But only 12% of the 2,503 persons 65 and older polled said loneliness was "very serious," compared with 7% of the under 65 group who reported the same problem.

Feeling needed: A 56% majority of all younger persons think that "not feeling needed is a very serious problem" for persons 65 and over. But only 7% of the elderly complain about not being needed, hardly more than the 5% of young persons who feel this way.

Poor health: Half of the younger group think that "poor health is a very serious" problem for those 65 and over, compared with 21% of the elderly who say health is one of their main problems. And 10% of the younger persons also suffer from chronic poor health.

This Harris Poll monograph has really upset many gerontologists, because everything is not as terrible for the aged as we professionals had wanted to believe. The picture that emerges is one of a group of people who have adequate self-esteem and who were coping well with problems of health, money, and crime, and who maintained frequent social contacts with a variety of role partners. There must be much more that is worthy of publication in the accumulated data tapes (Kalish, 1975).

We can learn from these few examples the importance of a control group and of selecting a random sample of older people. People who work with the aged in noninstitutional and even more so in institutional settings see a very small proportion of the aged. Many fewer than 10% of the aged participate in any age-segregated activity (Morris, 1969). As Tobin and Thompson (1975) have earlier demonstrated, these groups are almost always biased in some way or other. All professionals have a distorted view of the population: policemen deal with family conflict, alcohol problems, and crime (probably in that order of frequency) and see the population through those distorting lenses; physicians see sick people and the "worried well," and gerontologists see "problem" old people. But when one gets a bird's-eye view of the totality of old people by proper randomization of a sample (that is, of sampling all sections and groups of aged through using an appropriate methodology) and *compares old people with a representative sample of the nonaged*, the popular stereotypes disappear or their intensity is attenuated.

The Aged and Stressful Life Events

Life Change. It has often been hypothesized that life changes lead to illness. The school of Holmes, Rahe, Mesuda, et al., has developed scales of supposedly stressful life events that predispose to development of illness (Holmes and Rahe, 1967, especially refs. 2–8). Boyd and Oakes (1973) presented the position that, if this is the case, then older people must be at a greater risk, since they adapt less well than younger people to physiological stress. The relationship between stress and illness has been widely questioned for, among other reasons, employing crude analytic techniques (Rabkin and Struening, 1976); the enthusiasm of the devotees of life stress as *the* cause of illness is such that they have ignored such obvious non-psychological-stress causes of illness as jobs that bring workers into contact with swinging booms and scalding steam (Rubin et al., 1969); indeed, Holmes himself after a lecture in Birmingham blithely told me that our study of eighty-eight consecutive patients admitted to the Birmingham Veteran's Administration (VA) Hospital by medical residents not noted for their sympathy to the chronically ill, marginally employable, or unemployable older males (who percolate down to the VA hospital system as they become ineligible for or cannot afford private insurance) (Wershow and Reinhart, 1974), "proved (to Holmes at least) that these patients were not really sick." What else? Since the changes in their lives were practically nil, they had to be healthy, despite acute exacerbations of chronic kidney, lung, liver disease, ulcers, coronaries, and other severe medical problems that made admission to the VA hospital necessary. Since the facts didn't fit the theory, the facts had to be wrong! Yet "stressful life events account for only about 3 to 4% of the explained variance in illness" (Lin et al., 1979, p. 109). It is time for the professional journals to refuse to print such nonsense as a paper "proving" that hospitalization for coronary infarcts, in Finland, is "caused" by such minor stresses as twenty-five or thirty points on the scales used (Rahe et al., 1973) or the equivalent of receiving a traffic ticket during a vacation or during Christmas. It is preposterous to assert that a change in life score units (LCU) of from 16 to 22 has significant causal connection with life-threatening illness: not when the change to a more responsible job counts for 29 LCU and retirement for 40 LCU. We know that most people who do not retire because of illness manage to survive, and the evidence for increased morbidity after retirement is at best equivocal.

Let us admit that different individuals respond to stress in various ways other than by becoming ill, such as withdrawing from the field by sleep, denial, or other ways. Some even find constructive ways of dealing with changes. Similarly factors leading to illness have multiple paths of causation, including the virulence of the microbial or other agent, the physiological status of the host, and just plain luck, among others. It is no wonder that stressful events account for such a small portion of the explained variance in illness.

Relocation trauma. The other area of concern about response of the aged to stress deals with the phenomenon known as "relocation trauma." It is commonly believed that moving elderly people, especially into an institution for the aged, leads to heightened chance of mortality for the group. The approach is a limited one. Lieberman points out (1974), a point seconded by Borup et al. (1979), that "simply keeping the elderly alive, when our goal is to enhance service and the state of human beings . . . does not provide a meaningful approach to the problem" (p. 500). Preventing the absolute failure of death is not the same as ensuring a successful relocation. Lieberman notes that "relocation entails a higher than acceptable risk to the large majority of those being moved" (p. 495) such risk being defined as "marked decline, behaviorally, physically (including death), socially or psychologically . . . most individuals who are classified as marked decline showing multiple signs of such decline" (p. 495). Older people in bad states of physical functioning and cognitive ability, who feel despair and the inability to control their environment, and/or who employ primitive defense mechanisms such as denial are those most likely to decline following relocation; yet these are the very people who are most likely to require a highly supportive "prosthetic" environment. Lieberman studied elderly in four different kinds of environments prior to relocation, ranging from healthy elderly moving into "plush" institutions to the mass relocation of long-term state hospital inmates into whatever alternatives can be found (à la the problem earlier noted by Donahue, 1978). The elegance of Lieberman's conclusions on the characteristics of those who decline coming from and to various kinds of institutions is too detailed for this presentation. We deliberately omit the findings about the influence of the characteristics of the institutions (which are not irrelevant to outcomes) except to note that

> institutions that had relatively high expectational sets for behavior, that treated the elderly as adults with responsibilities, and that were not indulgent or permissive with regard to deviant behavior, presented a facilitative challenge. . . . (p. 500)
>
> Making demands in the context of a humanizing, respectful environment appears to be highly facilitative. Tender-loving-care when it implies infantilization seems . . . potentially destructive. In general, the call heard so frequently to make our institutions for the elderly

less total institutions does find support in our research. (Lieberman, 1974, p. 232)

This study echoes the findings of Blenkner et al. (1971), which discovered that elderly patients who received the full treatment of a protective service for the aged had higher rates of institutionalization and death than unserved controls in presumably equal need of service.

A recent paper by Borup et al. (1979), contrary to Lieberman, concludes categorically that the stress of "relocation does not bring about an increase in mortality" (p. 138). Borup does not consider the other, less absolute, losses that may accompany relocation; he notes in passing that we might do well "to focus on factors which would tend to extend the life of the elderly patient" (p. 139). His paper summarized the findings of twenty studies in addition to his own, which followed 529 patients in thirty nursing homes in Utah that were closed in 1974, following enforcement of stricter licensing laws, and compared them with a control group of 453 patients in nineteen nursing homes that remained open. Both Borup's study and 75% of the other twenty found no increase in death rates following relocation (the results of two studies were equivocal; some groups had higher death rates, others were unchanged). Borup properly questions the accuracy and consistency of record-keeping and changes in policies during periods of study of nursing homes toward admitting patients of differing health status, discharging moribund patients to die in hospitals, and other uncontrollable shifts, which constantly occur, to the despair of investigators, in many kinds of ongoing studies. Our own research (Wershow, 1976) shows that deaths in nursing homes, at least in Alabama, are so phenomenally high (44% within a month after admission) that increases could hardly be imagined.

This brief review evidences that the problem of "relocation trauma" is far from a settled issue in that (1) there is some question if it exists to an extent that measurable increase in deaths (if not other types of decline) are due to relocation, and (2) even if it is so proven, that much can be done about it, since those presumptively at highest risk are precisely those who require maximum care and who can least satisfactorily be dealt with in settings other than those giving (not offering) the most total, all-enveloping care.

Medically Unproven Therapies

Orthodox medical treatment as well as more heterodox and even outright quack treatments have their cycles of popularity. Emerson (1977) gives an excellent review of some treatments in the past, all of which are now regarded rather sheepishly by the medical profession. The "natural history" of a treatment follows a regular course (Peterson, 1978): it is at first accepted slowly; its use accelerates rapidly and becomes uncritically overenthusiastic; as deleterious side effects and even negative effects become evident, the treatment is then employed more conservatively. Its use may even be abandoned. This was standard practice in the use of new drugs before the introduction, after World War II, of randomized clinical trials. Such has been the case, not alone with medical therapies such as bland diets and milk for ulcers, which are totally ineffective, though still used, and soft diets for spastic colon (Sleisenger and Fordtran, 1978), but also with surgical interventions. Gastric freezing has been abandoned as a treatment for duodenal ulcer and it now seems that, not only is classical radical mastectomy plus radiation not likely to affect the outcome of the disease, but these treatments may make things worse (McPherson and Fox, 1977). Standard practices in medicine, which have had long and unquestioned use, when tested under controlled conditions, often prove worthless. To take several examples from a small area of medical practice, the treatment of digestive discomfort: Stress seems to be unrelated to ulcers and has been reported for only 0.4 to 1.4% of the Viet Nam casualties. Even under the enormous stress and distress of massive burns, ulcers rarely develop; bland diets do not reduce gastric activity after meals; milk is not only useless in the treatment of ulcers, it turns out to be a potent stimulus of acid secretion. In the treatment of irritable bowel syndrome, neither the traditional low residue diet nor the recently revived fad of high roughage diet has been proven effective in controlled clinical trials, though it seems that roughage is not harmful to most patients (Sleisenger and Fordtran, 1978); roughage may be useful in the prevention of diverticulitis disease of the colon, but not much else. Even the $500+ per day coronary intensive care unit doesn't seem to influence the mortality in heart attacks (Peterson, 1978). How much less faith may one have in less orthodox treatment? We will not discuss such issues as laetrile or megavitamin therapy (Herbert, 1978), which affect all age groups. As to laetrile, we need merely remind the young that we have been through that before; earlier the miracle drug that nasty physicians were keeping from the sufferers was krebiozin (Holland, 1966). We went through the same politically forced scientific investigation of an ineffective quack therapy, which proved, to nobody's surprise, to be useless. There are equal humbugs in treatment of aging, notably the procaine (GeroVital GH-3) treatment used mainly in Rumania; European travel agents sell packaged deals, transportation, treatment, and tour, which enrich the coffers of the Rumanian Democratic Socialist Republic, to what avail? A recent review of 285 articles and books, covering more than a hundred thousand patients, spanning a quarter century, concludes:

> This review of the literature yields no convincing evidence that, except for a possible anti-depressant effect, the systemic use of procaine (or GeroVital, of which the major component is procaine) is of value in the treatment of diseases in older patients. (Ostfeld et al., 1977, p. 16).

Nutrition Fads

The aged are more likely to be victims of health faddists and quacks because of generally lower education, chronic illness, and disability compounded by poverty and exacerbated (for some) by a fear of aging. All this makes them vulnerable to cheap and easy methods of dealing with physical concomitants of aging. Scientists strive for immortality by swallowing tales of very old people living somewhere else; lay people reach for a vitamin pill.

We need not dwell long on the foibles of the food faddists and megavitamin nuts. Deutsch (1977) and the American Psychiatric Association (1973) have done that most adequately. The popular belief is that, if X amount of vitamin, protein, or mineral is good for you, then 2X, 3X . . . will be 2, 3, or . . . times better. Indeed, excess of the fat-soluble vitamins (A and D) can be dangerous, causing for vitamin A, enlarged liver and spleen, increased intracranial pressure, irritability, and headache, and, for vitamin D, decreased appetite, nausea, weakness, weight loss, kidney stones, calcification of tissues, high blood pressure, and kidney failure leading to death. Vitamin E, which may improve sexual vigor in rats, *decreases* human sexual function and has no discernible positive effect on the human body. Excessive intake may lead to nausea, giddiness, headache, inflammation of the mouth and lips, and increased bleeding tendency. It also interferes with bodily absorption of vitamin C, which, highly touted as a preventive measure against colds, has no such effect, though it may reduce the severity of mild colds. Vitamin C also destroys vitamin B_{12}, and in large amounts produces diarrhea and kidney problems (Herbert, 1978; Barrett and Knight, 1976). As for "organically grown" foods—first, there is no control for the veracity of the claim that they are grown without pesticides (unless the fruits and vegetables are wormy), and use "natural" fertilizer (that is, manure). Animals that eat grasses grown on soil deficient in various trace minerals cannot return to that soil what they never imbibed. In addition, in the less developed countries whose peasants use organic wastes (including human wastes), intestinal parasitic diseases are endemic.

Part of the problem with dietary fads is that some people with excellent academic credentials promote these useless, expensive therapies, despite the total lack of evidence for their efficacy. No more than 2–3% of the elderly have overt nutritional deficiencies. Subclinical deficiencies, which may be evidenced by general malaise, weakness, and lethargy, are probably more prevalent but are difficult to document, as so many other conditions present the same symptoms, ranging from slowly growing bleeding cancers to simple depression. Old people are most likely (the third that does not consume an adequate diet) to be lacking in calcium (which may be the result of malabsorption), iron, and vitamins A and C (Harmon, 1979). These deficiencies are better and usually more cheaply remedied by better dentures, use of less expensive powdered low-fat milk, and green and yellow vegetables than by overdoses of expensive, potentially dangerous vitamins (which are even more expensive if they are "natural," made from rose hips and such, than if synthesized).

Psychosocial Therapies

Let us refer to the findings of Blenkner et al. (1971), mentioned earlier. In that study, an experimental group of confused aged in need of protective services (that is, guidance in spending money, protection against predatory neighbors, enlisting the support of family and friends) who were treated with "social therapies" did not differ in results from an untreated control group, except that the death rate of the experimental group was *higher!* The experimental group did have an improved physical environment (if one considers a larger proportion in a nursing home superior to coping with extrainstitutional living, however inadequate), received more services, and their families, at least, experienced less stress. The last was probably the effect of caseworkers teaching families better techniques for coping with their brain-damaged elders and helping the families to experience less guilt. There was, however, no effect on physical or mental functioning or contentment. In another study, Blenkner (1964) conducted a demonstration project providing concentrated service to the aged by public health nurses and social workers and learned that short-term treatment was better than long-term. This probably occurred because the teams, being unable to alleviate the situations of the elderly clients, which appeared appalling to the treatment personnel, relied heavily on institutional care, "which may actually accelerate decline". These studies are additional examples of therapeutic omnipotence referred to in discussing organic brain syndrome. If psychosocial therapies limited themselves to problems that had solutions, they may have a degree of success. Therapies may help people to better cope with limited problems such as life readjustment necessitated by a heart attack or loss of a spouse. They cannot, in and of themselves, deal with overwhelming problems such as living in a community despite a failing mind or in solving severe and chronic maladjustments by an hour or two a week of psychotherapy. Indeed, Fisher (1973a, 1973b, 1976) and Lieberman and Mullan (1978) question whether professional psychological help does anything at all for any patients and clients and their evidence is strong, if not wholly conclusive to those of us who have been on one or the other side of professional psychotherapeutic relationships.

Why are quack treatments so popular? First of all, there is a placebo effect, that is, the effect of strong belief by the patient and physician that the treatment is effective. Secondly, take any people away from their normal routines, subject them to the healthful routine of country air, a sensible diet, away from the usual pressure of their home environment, telephones, news, and TV, and the patients will usually feel better. That is the secret of success of any health spa! Thirdly, even the chronic illnesses of aging have their ups and downs and if the remission coincides with the useless treatment, that gets the credit.

In the "rules" stated in the introduction, we insisted on controlled, if possible double-blinded studies, before determining efficacy of any treatment. Anyone, scientist or not, who has spent several years developing a cure for a disease (or a better carburetor) has invested a great deal; he or she has a stake in the outcome. One's mind plays tricks on one in such circumstances. It is necessary to have as objective a standard as is possible to evaluate success or failure; the best standard is then properly tested by a double-blinded study, that is, the persons administering the therapy and/or evaluating the treatment do not know which patient is receiving the old treatment (or the placebo) and which the new. Only after the experiment is finished is it revealed which patient got which treatment; thereby everybody is guarded against both conscious and unconscious biases. No drug therapy can be considered adequate by any other test of its efficacy (Di Palma, 1976).

Whatever the problems of evaluating medical treatment, the problems of evaluating psychosocial treatment are staggering.

Recommended Readings

Deutsch, R. *The New Nuts Among the Berries*. Palo Alto: Bull Publishing Co., 1977.

Fisher, J. *The Effectiveness of Social Casework*. Springfield, Ill.: Charles C Thomas, 1976.

Harris, L. and Associates. "The Myth and Reality of Aging in America." Washington, D.C.: National Council on Aging, 1975.

Lieberman, M. and Mullun, J. "Does Help Help? The Adaptive Consequences of Obtaining Help from Professionals and Social Networks." *American Journal of Community Psychology* 6 (499–517):1978.

Rabkin, J. and Struening, E. "Life Events, Stress and Illness." *Science* 194 (1976):1013–20.

The controversy over *relocation trauma* is continued in two articles in *The Gerontologist*, 21 (February 1981), "The effects of relocation on the elderly: a reply to Borup, J. H., Gallego, D. T., and Hefferran, P. G." by N. Boureston and Leon Pastalan, pp. 4–7 and "Mortality as affected by interinstitutional relocation: update and assessment" by J. H. Borup and D. T. Gallego, pp. 8–16.

Part Seven
Epilogue

13

Toward a Philosophy of Mature Aging

The Indian Summer of life should be a little sunny and a little sad, like the season.

Henry Adams, *The Education of Henry Adams*

Editor's Introduction

The compiler of this anthology hopes that readers will see it, not as the expression of a negative attitude toward the old and the study of aging, but rather as a clearing of the air of much misconception, fuzzy thinking and false sentimentality. The following paper sums up what I consider to be the spirit of this volume. Kalish's polemic brings into sharp focus many of the conflicts that arise out of the struggle between gerontology as a field of scientific endeavor and gerontology as a cause. When the need to serve the cause outdistances the limits of scientific knowledge and optimism goes beyond the limits of reality, gerontologists and gerontology both get into trouble. Kalish, in this essay and elsewhere, stands on solid scientific and humanistic ground. Not everything we do or advocate requires a solid scientific base. There is, for example, no need to "prove" that adequate nutrition prolongs life, mental alertness, physical fitness, sexual power, or anything else. In this country, at least, every human being can be adequately fed and as long as this is possible, nobody should go hungry. No members of any group should be without provision of services, wherever these can be provided.

Our editorial comments must end on that note.

The New Ageism and the Failure Models: A Polemic

R. A. Kalish

Social gerontologists and social geriatricians have made considerable use of the term *ageism* as a counterpart to the more familiar *racism* and *sexism*. The general assumption underlying the application of this term is that ageist individuals and ageist societies or communities or organizations exist.

Ageists, the assumption holds, express overt and covert dislike and discrimination regarding the elderly. That is, they avoid older persons on an individual level, they discriminate against older persons in terms of jobs, other forms of access to financial support, utilization of social institutions, and so forth. Further, the ageist individual derides the elderly through hostile humor, through accusations that the elderly are largely responsible for their own plight, and through complaints that they are consuming more than their share of some particular resource. They may also contend that older people deserve what they get, are in effect a drain on society, are functionally incapable of change or improvement (or, conversely, are capable of change and improvement and should be required to do so with their present resources), and do not contribute adequately to the society from which they are taking resources. Ageism involves stereotyping, prejudice, discrimination, segregation, hostility . . . the list can go on and on.

The New Ageism

I would like to propose that there is another form of ageism, that it is equally pervasive in our society, and that it is found in advocates of the elderly as often—and perhaps more so—than among their antagonists.

This form of ageism, which I will refer to as the New Ageism, although it is certainly not new, has the following characteristics:

(1) It stereotypes "the elderly" in terms of the characteristics of the least capable, least healthy, and least alert of the elderly, although its rhetoric is punctuated by insistence that "all elderly are not alike."

(2) It perceives the older person as, in effect, a relatively helpless and dependent individual who requires the support services of agencies and other organizations.

(3) It encourages the development of services without adequate concern as to whether the outcome of these services contributes to reduc-

tion of freedom for the participants to make decisions controlling their own lives.

(4)   It produces an unrelenting stream of criticism against society in general and certain individuals in society for their mistreatment of the elderly, emphasizing the unpleasant existence faced by the elderly.

The message of the New Ageism seems to be that "we" understand how badly you are being treated, that "we" have the tools to improve your treatment, and that if you adhere to our program, "we" will make your life considerably better. You are poor, lonely, weak, incompetent, ineffectual, and no longer terribly bright. You are sick, in need of better housing and transportation and nutrition, and we—the nonelderly and those elderly who align themselves with us and work with us—are finally going to turn our attention to you, the deserving elderly, and relieve your suffering from ageism.

The New Ageism obscures individual and group differences within the 23,000,000 or so persons in the country normally defined as elderly. In fact, the definition of "elderly" tends to slip and slide a bit, which permits the New Ageists to seem on more solid ground than they really are. The New Ageists begin by stating that there are 23,000,000 persons over age 65; they often ignore the immense diversity among these persons and they also tend to ignore that most of these persons are intact, functioning effectively on their own, and getting along adequately on what money they have. Then their definition of "the elderly" changes from one based on chronological age to one based on sickness and poverty, but the change is implicit, not explicit, and so the listener is still focused on the 23,000,000 elderly and makes the assumption, without realizing it, that the spotlighted elderly represent the totality of elderly.

The Failure Models

The New Ageism has another message, one which I believe is more subtle and more pervasive than the message described in the previous discussion: the Failure Models. The general message of the Failure Models is that this or that older person has failed or is going to fail. This is accomplished in two related but very different fashions: the Incompetence Model, an approach that constantly reminds older people how incompetent they are; and the Geriactivist Model, an approach that establishes a rigid set of standards for appropriate behavior and faults those who do not adhere to the standards.

The Incompetence Failure Model has been developed in part as a tactic to get funding from governmental and private agencies. In effect, it is the ability to say, "Those persons for whom I am advocate are greater failures than those persons for whom you are advocate. They are such great failures that the only solution to their failure is more money." The obvious difficulty with this model is that as soon as the failures become successes, the incompetents become competent and in need of fewer services, and the advocates will lose their jobs and, more than that, lose their status as serving the "Incompetent Failure of the Year."

This model is best represented by a superficial reading of the distressingly excellent Pulitzer Prize winning book, *Why Survive?*, by Robert Butler. I describe this as "best" because it simultaneously is a masterful job of chronicling the ills that have befallen the elderly, basing this chronicle on thorough research and careful documentation, and includes a virtually prototypical example of the Incompetence Failure Model. This book has served effectively to rally the sympathetic and persuade the dubious that the plight of the elderly requires remediation. But what accumulative effect does this book, and its kindred media and political writings and speeches, have on older persons? Now that television and columnists have "discovered" the elderly, how has their discovery affected the persons discovered?

I certainly admit that I don't know these answers; indeed I don't think that anyone has a clear idea. There are no research data, and I cannot recall ever having read any analytical article. The very title of Butler's book suggests a possible reaction that an elderly reader or, even more likely, a reader approaching his or her later years, would have: Why Survive? Indeed, what can be gained by living?

One possible effect on older people of the Incompetence Failure Model is that they internalize what they read and hear and come to believe it of themselves as individuals. If this is the case, then the work of the advocates of the elderly becomes as damaging to the self-esteem of older persons as is the view of those who damn them with benign neglect or even those who express overt ageism.

A second possibility is that each older individual accepts the information literally, but excludes himself or herself and closer friends. This is the "those-old-people-over-there" position. A third alternative is that the rhetoric and polemic are seen as political in nature and have little or no effect at all. And a fourth is that the elderly individual is strengthened by recognizing the responsibility for his or her plight as emanating from a society that ignores him or her, thus requiring a redoubling of effort which will lead to the assuaging of discomfort.

I suspect that all of these operate, at different times and with different persons, although I believe that the second view prevails. Thus, the elderly person denies that the model applies to him or her, but acknowledges that it is descriptive of "those old folks."

I don't wish to make a scapegoat of *Why Survive?* It served a very important purpose, but unfortunately the valuable discussion of a better life for the elderly in the later part of the book did not receive the attention that the earlier Incompetence Failure Model received. Nor do I wish to present the position that the elderly need all kinds of protection. That notion has been exaggerated: the elderly are much tougher and more resilient than they are given credit for being.

The second message of failure is the Geriactivist Model. I coined this term about ten years ago to describe the older people who are themselves active in the causes of the elderly. They develop a symbiotic relationship with younger advocates, and together they maintain the call for an active and involved old age. The Geriactivist needs the younger associates who have jobs in the community and who can participate in making decisions; the younger advocates—social workers, recreation workers, agency staff, politicians—need the activist older person as both a source of inexpensive support labor and to legitimize the activist position. The activist position is established as the *only* appropriate way for older persons to function. Something is assumed to be wrong with older people who wish to sit around and talk with elderly friends, who wish to stay at home and read, who thoroughly enjoy television, who wish to pray or meditate or jog by themselves, who for whatever reasons prefer their world to be comfortable, comforting, and manageable rather than stimulating, challenging, and risky, who prefer their inner worlds to the external world. One geriactivist—my model for this role—went so far as to tell me that any older person who would not participate actively, either socially or politically, was probably lacking in moral integrity or in emotional stability.

Older persons who respond to their inner worlds or who enjoy and desire passive entertainment are seen as challenges to be overcome, rather than as individuals who are adapting to a life-long (or recent) preference that could only be fully realized when retirement and the empty nest made it possible. Thus, once again the sense of failure is communicated. "Those who are not part of the solution are part of the problem; those who do not adhere to my rules of healthy old age are, by definition, failures." Diversity is not recognized, nor are inner life and intrinsic satisfactions seen as a proper definition for a healthy personality.

Overall the Failure Models probably generate anger among the elderly with society and simultaneously with themselves. The implication is that the older person is not only victimized, but also is impotent and powerless to have any significant impact on the society and/or individuals who perpetrate the victimization. The built-in assumption is that change is governed from without, a view guaranteed to intensify the sense of impotence. And since the older person is perceived by others through the lens of this model, the initial response many people have to the older person is that of helpless victim, a view made worse by the assumption that it actually favors the elderly.

The source of the victimization is often stated as being an impersonal bureaucracy and a depersonalizing society, run for the betterment of some vaguely labeled "establishment" or else for some other age or power group. All of this adds up to a perceived conspiracy to deprive the elderly of their entitlements, a situation guaranteed to increase frustration and anger. And made worse by the pity and sympathy that are often the result. Further, to the extent that it is perceived as accurate and authoritative, it will discourage older persons from attempts to gain their rights since this will be seen as a futile action.

Perpetrators or Innocent Bystanders?

Who is really responsible for the Failure Models? Is it the funding agencies that must compete with other funding agencies in their presentation to Congress of the dire need they represent? Perhaps, but only in part, since it is obviously political pressure, as well as extent of need, that produces results.

Are the media responsible? Yes and no. Certainly they exploit the Failure Models, but nonetheless they tend to respond primarily to what they perceive their audience as wanting to view.

Are the members of Congress the true villains? No, since they only respond to some combination of political demand and perceived need.

Is it we gerontologists and geriatricians? Again, yes and no. We are familiar with the successes, and we are familiar with the need to respect diversity, but we are also pressured by the importance of keeping our own programs going, and we can't do this without money and personal support. At the same time, many of us are both active and activists, and our natural inclination is to view these qualities in others in a positive light. Indeed, for some of us, our entire professional value system is predicated on the importance of activity and involvement. What is important to watch here is how we define involvement and that we do not place highly restrictive boundaries on what we consider mentally healthy aging.

So who has perpetrated the Failure Models? All of us, and with many valid reasons, but without adequate thought of consequences. There was a time in history when people who succeeded were considered to be chosen by God, when it was often assumed that those who were healthy or financially successful must be so because of God's will. Now the opposite view seems to prevail, and advocates focus on the weaknesses and victimization of those they represent in order to develop a viable position.

There are no villians, yet we are all responsible.

Some Existing Models and an Alternative

In the 15 or so years that I have been involved in gerontology, I have noted several models in our society that have been used to describe the nature of aging. I'm presenting them here, fully cognizant that they are highly impressionistic and far from being expressed in readily operational terms.

The first model I've termed the Pathology Model. Old age is seen as pathological, a time of sickness and strangeness and falling-apartness. It is also seen as a static period, without much chance for change in a positive direction. It just *is*.

Following that, both in severity and, in my experience, in chronology, is the Decrement Model. This model is based on cross-sectional studies that showed the substantial age-related differences that were initially interpreted as age-related changes. Decrements are not as bad as pathology, but they partake of the same kind of distress.

The third model, initiated when we became aware that longitudinal studies suggested a much smaller decrement than previously assumed, might be termed the Minimal Change Model. Herein older people were presumed to be continuations of what they were as younger people, but with a small degree of decrement. So we talked about biochemical and social and psychological and health impairments that could occur at any age, but occurred more frequently with old age and are sometimes accumulative so that they were, in any event, likely to take a heavier toll in the later years. In these ways, age per se was not the villain, but the age-related changes were.

The fourth model prevails among gerontologists today. It is the Normal Person Model. Older people are simply people, like all other individuals. They are highly diverse. They do resemble each other in some ways, because of when they were socialized to certain values or when they experienced certain events; they share increased likelihood of being grandparents, being retired, being diabetic, being widowed, but they differ in more ways than they are similar. Their behavior is understandable in terms of the situations they confront, so that any form of conservatism is explained in terms of their social and political values and the economic situation they face; reaction time changes are explained in terms of biochemical changes that the elderly learn to compensate for with considerable success; cognitive changes are likely to arise from isolation as often as from physiological brain change, but in either event, it is a health problem, not an aging problem per se.

I would like to propose a fifth model, perhaps an outgrowth of the Normal Person Model: a Personal Growth model. The later years can be a period of optimum personal growth. Not for everyone: some are not in adequate health, some are too financially restricted, some have been socialized in their early years in ways of thinking and behaving that make later growth impossible. But the later years can be a time for growth. For one thing, many earlier responsibilities are no longer in evidence. Children no longer make significant demands; aged parents are often (but not always) dead; repetitive and unstimulating jobs no longer consume time and energy; stressful competitive needs no longer stir the ego.

Second, older persons no longer need to be constrained by what others think of them. No longer are they likely to be threatened with loss of jobs or the demands of dependent children if they step outside the fences that had previously circled their lives. Of course, they may not be able to do this, or they may not wish to do this, but the option is there.

Third, many elderly have worked through their fears of their own death, and they have therefore learned better than any others how to develop priorities that satisfy them. They have also learned to cope with their own health problems and with losing others. Obviously, death, health, and loss don't cease to be problems, but many older persons have a period of years—sometimes many years—when these are not inhibiting problems.

Fourth, there is tremendous discretionary time. One of the major difficulties of retirement is that of using time for one's own satisfaction. Those who fail to solve this problem probably do not lead enjoyable retirement lives; those who do solve the problem learn how to schedule themselves for optimum pleasure, whether the pleasure comes through physical labor, social relationships, or leisure.

Fifth, there is the motivation caused by knowing the future is finite. For some elderly, this knowledge is so destructive that enjoyment or satisfaction is virtually impossible. Others, however, not only cope more effectively, but respond to the pressure by a highly appropriate use of time. The time boundary justifies their ignoring the minutes of life, if they wish, and to concentrate on what matters to them. This might be gardening or painting or political action or earning money or seeking enlightenment or praying or talking with friends or reminiscing. They do not mark time; they use time for themselves. They learn to enjoy the passing minutes by becoming absorbed in those minutes.

The Personal Growth Model of aging is obviously not one I have created in this paper. The SAGE program, developed by Gay Luce, has been using this model for several years; many senior centers have encouraged personal growth; the rapidly increasing emphasis on facilitating the return of older people to formal and informal educational programs reflects the same intent. Nonetheless, there is too little awareness of the potential for continued growth and personal satisfaction among the elderly and, simultaneously, unduly narrow boundaries as to what constitutes growth and satisfaction.

Some Final Preaching

I am not Pollyanna. Normally I am Cassandra. I do not wish to take a Geriactivist position and place the burden of trying to attain a standard of personal growth on an elderly person who is fighting for life against physical or financial hardship. Rather, I am trying to emphasize the possibility of growth at any time in life and the recognition that the growth that does not occur in the later years is never going to occur.

I am also suggesting that we can develop a Personal Growth model, so that we approach older persons with the expectation that they have the potential for continued growth, that even sickness and financial restriction can be a source of growth, although not desirable, and that our task is to facilitate that growth.

There are programs, many programs, that are doing just that, and there are articles in the media and television programs that show what these programs are doing. Often, of course, the implication of the media is that these older people are unusual and that is why we must put them on display, but the other message can also be heard: you too can be like these people.

There is also something that each individual can do, rather than feeling helpless to fight the overpowering bureaucracy. We can communicate to older persons that we have faith in their abilities, that we recognize that they are capable of making decisions (even those decisions that we assume, perhaps correctly, will turn out wrong), that we respect their ownership of their own bodies and time and lives. In brief, we can communicate a Success Model instead of the Failure Models.

It is not my point that the elderly in the U.S. and Canada enjoy the best in the best of all possible countries. Many older people are certainly in need of better housing, better transportation systems, better nutrition, more recognition of needs for human relationships and for stimulation and challenges. Nor is this a call for reduced services. Needs and wants will always outrun resources.

The difficulty is that by describing the elderly as helpless individuals, beset by problems, incompetent in finding their own ways, and obligated to meet a set standard of activity, we are expressing the New Ageism. It influences our views of the elderly, their view of themselves, and—I can only assume—the behavior that both the elderly and nonelderly exhibit in regard to aging and older people. If we define older people as victims, we will approach them as victims and expect them to behave as victims. Even by defining something as A Problem, we are initiating a self-fulfilling prophecy.

I would like to see the definition of older people develop so that they are perceived as equally—perhaps more—capable of personal growth and life satisfaction and happiness. This means a Success Model instead of a Failure Model, without blinding us to the very real problems that some older people do face. We can then stop confusing the elderly with the least competent consumers of geriatric services, and begin to work toward the development of a community that recognizes the competent, autonomous, self-esteeming, generative older person as the norm. We can refocus our attention on the later years as opportunities for flexibility, joy, pleasure, growth, and sensuality.

Recommended Readings

Berl, F. "Growing Up to Old Age." *Social Work* 8 (1963):85–91.

Coles, R. *The Old Ones of New Mexico*. New York: Anchor Books, 1975.

Havice, D. "Old Age: The Possibility of Enlightenment." *Soundings* (Spring, 1974):70–79.

Saul, S. *Aging: An Album of People Growing Old*. New York: Wiley, 1974.

References

Adams, R. and Smith, T. *Fear of Neighborhood*. Chicago: National Opinion Research Center Report 127 e, forthcoming.

Ahern, D. "Social Security—A Gross Misnomer, Especially for Women." *Prime Time* 2 (January 1974):11–14.

Alikishiev, P. "Longevity in Dagestan." In *Problems of Gerontology*, edited by V. Alpatov. Moscow: Academy of Sciences of USSR, 1962.

American Psychiatric Association. *Megavitamin and Orthomolecular Therapy in Psychiatry*. Washington: American Psychiatric Association, 1973.

Anderson, O. "Reflections on the Sick Aged and the Helping Systems." In *Social Policy, Social Ethics, and the Aging Society*, edited by B. Neugarten and R. Havighurst. Washington, D.C.: National Science Foundation, 1976.

Anderson, F. and Carlton-Ashton, J., eds. "Brain Failure in Old Age." *Age and Ageing* (Supplementary Issue) 6 (1977).

Anonymous. "Case Conference . . . Strive Officiously to Keep Alive." *Journal of Medical Ethics* 3 (1977):189–73.

Antunes, G.; Cook, F.; Cook, T.; and Skogan, W. "Patterns of Personal Crimes Against the Elderly." *Gerontologist* 17 (1977):321–27.

Arie, T. "Thoughts on Rationing and Responsibility." In W. Anderson and J. Carlton-Ashton (Eds.) *Brain Failure in Old Age*. (*Age and Ageing* Supplementary Issue) 6 (1977):104–7.

Armstrong, P. "Comment: More Thoughts on Senility." *Gerontologist* 18 (1978):315–16.

Arnoff, C. "Old Age in Prime Time." *Journal of Communication* 24 (Autumn 1974):86–87.

Atchley, R. "Retirement and Leisure Participation: Continuity or Crisis?" *Gerontologist* 11 (1971):13–17.

———. *The Social Forces in Later Life: An Introduction to Social Gerontology*. Belmont, Calif.: Wadsworth, 1972.

Axinin, J. and Levin, H. *Social Welfare: A History of the American Response to Needs*. Philadelphia: University of Pennsylvania Press, 1975.

Baltes, P. B. "Longitudinal and Cross-Sectional Sequences in the Study of Aging and Generations Effect." *Human Development* 11 (1968):145–71.

Baltes, P. B. and Schaie, K. W. "Aging and IQ: The Myth of the Twilight Years." *Psychology Today* 7 (March 1974):35–40.

———. "On the Plasticity of Intelligence in Adulthood and Old Age: Where Horn and Donaldson Fail." *American Psychologist* 31 (1976):720–25.

Barrett, S. and Knight, G., eds. *The Health Robbers*. Philadelphia: George F. Stickley, 1976.

Bart, P. "Depression in Middle-aged Women." In *Women in Sexist Society*, edited by V. Gornick and B. Moran. New York: Basic Books, 1971.

Beeson, D. "Women in Studies of Aging: A Critique and Suggestion." *Social Problems* 23 (1975):52–59.

Benet, S. "Why They Live to be 100, or Even Older in Abkhasia." *New York Times Magazine*, 26 December 1971.

Benedict, R. *Patterns of Culture*. Boston: Houghton Mifflin, 1934.

Berdyshev G. "Possible Role of Heterosis for Longevity." In *Problems of Aging and Longevity*, edited by V. Meirek. Moscow: Nauka, 1966.

———. *Ecological and Genetic Factors of Aging and Longevity*. Leningrad: Nauka, 1968.

Berl, F. "Growing Up to Old Age." *Social Work* 8 (January 1963):85–91.

Berquist, L. "Recycling Lives." *Ms.*, August 1973, pp. 59–105.

Biddle, B. and Thomas, E., eds. *Role Theory: Concepts and Research*. New York: Wiley, 1966.

Binstock, R. "Interest-Group Liberalism and the Politics of Aging." *Gerontologist* 12 (1972):265–80.

———. "Federal Policy toward the Aged: Its Inadequacies and Its Politics." *National Journal*, 11 November 1978, pp. 1837–45.

Binstock, R. and Shanas, E., eds. *Handbook of Aging and the Social Sciences*. New York: Van Nostrand, 1976.

Birmingham News. "Teenager Dying of Cancer Welcomed to Waikiki." 17 February 1975.

Birren, J., ed. *Handbook of Aging and the Individual*. Chicago: University of Chicago Press, 1959.

Birren, J.; Greenhouse, S.; Sokaloff, L.; and Yarrow, M. *Human Aging: A Biological and Behavioral Study*. Bethesda, Md.: National Institute of Mental Health, 1963.

Blau, Z. *Old Age in a Changing Society*. New York: New Viewpoints, 1973.

Blazer, D. and Palmore, E. "Religion and Aging in a Longitudinal Panel." *Gerontologist* 16 (1976):82–85.

Blenkner, M.; Bloom, M.; and Nielsen, M. "A Research and Demonstration Project of Protective Services." *Social Casework* 52 (1971):483–500.

Blenkner, M.; Jahn, J.; and Wasser, E. *Serving the Aging, an Experiment in Social Work and Public Health Nursing*. New York: Community Service Society, 1964.

Bogomoletz, A., ed. *Aging*. Kiev: Ukranian Academy of Sciences, 1940.

Borup, J.; Gallego, D.; and Herman, P. "Relocation and Its Effect on Mortality." *Gerontologist* 19 (1979):135–40.

Botwinick, J. *Cognitive Processes in Maturity and Old Age*. New York: Springer, 1967.

———. "Intellectual Abilities." In *Handbook of the Psychology of Aging*, edited by J. Birren and W. Schaie. New York: Van Nostrand, 1977.

———. "Intelligence." In *Aging and Behavior*, edited by J. Botwinick. New York: Springer, 1978.

Boyd, R. and Oakes, C. *Foundations of Practical Gerontology*. 2d ed. Columbia, S.C.: University of South Carolina Press, 1973.

Brabec, B. "Being Our Age and Learning to Like It." *Prime Time* (January 1974):5–6.

Broberg, M.; Melching, D.; and Maeda, D. "Planning for the Elderly in Japan." *Gerontologist* 15 (1975):242–47.

Brocklehurst, J. "Brain Failure in Old Age: Social Implications." In W. Anderson and J. Carlton-Ashton (Eds.) *Brain Failure in Old Age*. (*Age and Ageing* Supplementary Issue) 6 (1977):30–34, 36–40, with discussion by Drs. Arie, Bergmann, Irvine, Middleton, and Robinson.

Brody, E.; Kleban, J.; Lawton, M.; and Silverman, H. "Excess Disability in the Aged: Impact of Individualized Treatment. *Gerontologist* 11 (1971):124–33.

Brody, E.; Cole, C.; and Moss, M. "Individualizing Therapy for the Mentally Impaired Aged." *Social Casework* 54 (1973):453–61.

Brody, E.; Kleban, M.; Lawton, M.; and Moss, M. "A Longitudinal Look at Excess Disabilities." *Journal of Gerontology* 29 (1974):79–84.

Brotman, H. "The Fastest Growing Minority: The Aged." *American Journal of Public Health* 64 (1974):251.

———. "Advanced Data on Income in 1975, with Revisions of Published Data for 1974." Washington, D.C.: U.S. Bureau of Census, 1976.

Brown, M. "Nurses' Attitudes toward the Aged and Their Care." *Annual Report to the Gerontology Branch*, USPHS. Washington, D.C.: U.S. Government Printing Office, 1967.

Bunker, J.; Barnes, B.; and Moesteller, F., eds. *Costs, Risks, and Benefits of Surgery*. London: Oxford University Press, 1977.

Busse, E. and Pfeiffer, E., eds. *Behavior and Adaptation in Late Life*. Boston: Little, Brown, 1977.

Butler, R. *Why Survive? Being Old in America*. New York: Harper & Row, 1975.

———. "Why Survive–2078?" Paper read at University of Minnesota Conference on Frontiers in Aging: Life Extension, 27 April 1978.

Butler, R., and Lewis, M. *Aging and Mental Health: Positive Psychological Approaches*. St. Louis: C. V. Mosby, 1973.

Caine, L. *Widow*. New York: William Morrow, 1974.

Campbell, M. "Study of the Attitudes of Nursing Personnel Toward the Geriatric Patient." *Nursing Research* 20 (1971):147–51.

Cannon, W. *Bodily Changes in Pain, Hunger, Fear, and Rage*. 2d ed. New York: Appleton, 1929.

Catholic Digest. "Survey of Religions in the U.S.", 7 (1966):27.

Cattell, R. "Are I.Q. Tests Intelligent?" *Psychology Today* 1 (March 1958):4–10.

Cavan, R. "Self and Role in Adjustment During Old Age." In *Human Behavior and Social Processes*, edited by A. Rose. Boston: Houghton Mifflin, 1962.

Chadwick, T. Review of E. Palmore, *The Honorable Elders*. *Gerontologist* 16 (1976):560–61.

Chaiffetz, M. Untitled article. *Gerontologist* 8 (1968):244.

Clemente, F. and Kleiman, M. "Fear of Crime among the Aged." *Gerontologist* 16 (1976):207–10.

Club of Rome. *The Limits of Growth*. Bloomfield, N.J.: University Press, 1972.

Coe, R. "Professional Perspectives on the Aged." *Gerontologist* 7 (1967):114–19.

Cohen, E. "Editorial: The Unseen Plague out of the Closet." *Gerontologist* 17 (1977):295, 302.

——. "Editorial: Teratogenesis and the Policy-Makers." *Gerontologist* 18 (1978):101.

Cohen, G. "Comment: Organic Brain Syndrome. Reality Orientation for Critics of Clinical Interventions." *Gerontologist* 18 (1978):313–14.

Comfort, A. "A Longer Life-Span by 1990?" *New Scientist* 44 (1969):545–55.

——. "We Know the Aging Process Can Be Slowed Down." In *The Center Eclectics*. Santa Barbara: Center for Study of Democratic Institutions, 1974.

Cook, T. and Campbell, D. *Quasi-Experimentation: Design and Analysis Issues for Field Settings*. Chicago: Rand McNally, 1979.

Cook, F. and Cook, T. "Evaluating the Rhetoric of Crisis: A Case Study of Criminal Victimization of the Elderly. *Social Service Review* 50 (1976):632–46.

——. "Criminal Victimization of the Elderly: Is the Crisis Rhetoric Warranted Yet?" Original contribution, 1979.

Cook, F.; Fremming, J.; and Tyler, T. "Criminal Victimization of the Elderly: Validating the Policy Assumptions." In *Progress in Applied Social Psychology*, edited by J. Davis and W. Stephenson. London: Wiley Europe, forthcoming.

Cook, F.; Skogan, W.; Cook, T.; and Antunes, G. "Criminal Victimization of the Elderly: The Physical and Economic Consequences." *Gerontologist* 18 (1978):338–49.

Cooper, B. and Piro, P. "Age Differences in Medical Care Spending, Fiscal Year 1973." *Social Security Bulletin* 37 (1974):3–14.

Cottrell, L. "The Adjustment of the Individual to His Age and Sex Roles." *American Sociological Review* 7 (1942):617–22.

Cowgill, D. and Holmes, L., eds. *Aging and Modernization*. New York: Appleton-Century-Crofts, 1972.

Cumming, E. "New Thoughts on the Theory of Disengagement." *International Social Science Journal* 15 (1963):337–93. Also in *New Thoughts on Old Age*, edited by R. Kastenbaum. New York: Springer, 1964.

——. "Engagement with an Old Theory." *Aging and Human Development* 6 (1975):247–51.

Cumming, E. and Henry, W. *Growing Old: The Process of Disengagement*. New York: Basic Books, 1961.

Cunningham, C. *The Pattern of Crime Against the Aging: The Kansas City Study*. (Paper presented at the National Conference on Crime Against the Elderly.) Washington, D.C.: U.S. Government Printing Office, 1975.

Cutler, S. and Kaufman R. "Cohort Changes in Political Attitudes." *Public Opinion Quarterly* 39 (1975):69–81.

Cyrus-Lutz, C. and Gaitz, C. "Psychiatrists' Attitudes toward the Aged and Aging." *Gerontologist* 12 (1972):163–67.

Dean, L. "Aging and Decline of Affect." *Journal of Gerontology* 17 (1962):440–46.

Decter, M. *The Liberated Woman and Other Americans*. New York: Coward, McCann & Geoghegan, 1971.

de Grazia, S. *Of Time, Work and Leisure*. New York: Anchor Books, 1964.

De Lora, J. and Moses, D. "Specialty Preferences and Characteristics of Nursing Students in Baccalaureate Programs." *Nursing Research* 18 (1969):137–44.

Demming, J. and Pressey, S. "Tests 'Indigenous' to the Adult and Older Years." *Journal of Counseling Psychology* 4 (1957):144–48.

Denes, M. *In Necessity and Sorrow: Life and Death in an Abortion Hospital*. New York: Basic Books, 1976.

de Schweinitz, K. *England's Road to Social Security*. Philadelphia: University of Pennsylvania Press, 1943.

Deutsch, R. *The New Nuts among the Berries*. Palo Alto: Bull Publishing Co., 1977.

Di Palma, J. "Basic Pharmacology in Medicine." In *Clinical Pharmacology*, Edited by J. Di Palma. New York: McGraw-Hill, 1976.

Dlin, B.; Stern, A.; and Poliakoff, S. "Survivors of Cardiac Arrest: The First Few Days." *Psychosomatics* 15 (1974):61–67.

Donahue, W. "What About Our Responsibility toward the Abandoned Elderly?" *Gerontologist* 18 (1978):102–11.

Dunkle, R. *Life Experience of Women and Old Age*. Paper presented at 25th annual meeting of Gerontological Society, San Juan, 17–21 December 1972.

Eisdorfer, C. and Lawton, M. eds. *The Psychology of Human Development and Aging*. Washington, D.C.: American Psychological Association, 1973.

Emerson, G., ed. *Aging*. Stroudsburg, Pa.: Dowden, Hutchinson and Ross, 1977.

Ennis, P. *Criminal Victimization in the United States: A Report of a National Survey*. National Opinion Research Center, University of Chicago. Washington, D.C.: U.S. Government Printing Office, 1967.

Epstein, L. and Murray, J. *The Aged Population of the United States*. Washington, D.C.: U.S. Government Printing Office, 1967.

Erskine, H. "The Polls." *Public Opinion Quarterly* 28 (1964):679.

Farber, L. "I'm Sorry, Dear." *Commentary* 38 (November 1964):47–54.

———. "Oh, Death, Where Is Thy Sting-a-ling-a-ling?" *Commentary* 63 (June 1977):35–43.

Feifel, H., ed. *The Meaning of Death*. New York: McGraw-Hill, 1959.

Fisher, J. "Is Casework Effective? A Review." *Social Work* 18 (January 1973a):5–20.

———. "Has Mighty Casework Struck Out?" *Social Work* 18 (July 1973b):107–10.

———. *The Effectiveness of Social Casework*. Springfield, Ill.: Charles C Thomas, 1976.

Flemming, A. "Flemming Urges Action in Crime Against the Elderly." *Aging* 250 (August 1975):4.

Ford, G. "Crime Message to Congress" (office of the White House Press Secretary, 19 June 1975), and "Remarks of the President to the California State Legislature" (office of the White House Press Secretary, 5 September 1975).

Forston, R. and Kitchens, J. *Criminal Victimization of the Aged: The Houston Model Neighborhood Area*. North Texas State University, 1974.

Fox, R. and Swaizey, J. *The Courage to Fail*. Chicago: University of Chicago Press, 1974.

Friday, P. "Sanctioning in Sweden: An Overview." *Federal Probation* 40 (September 1976):48–55.

Frolkis, V. "Mechanisms of Longevity." In *Gerontology and Geriatrics 1972 Year Book: Longevous People*, edited by D. Chebotarev. Kiev: Institute of Gerontology, 1973.

Fuchs, V. *Who Shall Live? Health, Economics and Social Choice*. New York: Basic Books, 1974.

Furry, C. and Baltes, P. "The Effect of Age Differences in Ability—Extraneous Performance Variables on the Assessment of Intelligence in Children, Adults and the Elderly." *Journal of Gerontology* 28 (1973):73–80.

Gale, J. and Livesley, B. "Attitudes toward Geriatrics: A Report of the King Survey." *Age and Ageing* 3 (1974):49–53.

Garfinkel, R. "The Reluctant Therapist." *Gerontologist* 15 (1975):136–37.

Gertz, M. and Talarico, S. "Problems of Reliability and Validity in Criminal Research." *Journal of Criminal Justice* 5 (Fall 1977):217–24.

Glenn, N. and Hefner, T. "Further Evidence on Aging and Party Identification." *Public Opinion Quarterly* 36 (1972):31–47.

Goddard, J. "Extension of the Lifespan: A National Goal?" In *Extending the Human Life Span: Social Policy and Social Ethics*, edited by B. Neugarten and R. Havighurst. Washington, D.C.: National Science Foundation, 1977.

Goldfarb, A. "The Rationale for Psychotherapy with Older People." *American Journal of Medical Sciences* 232 (1956):181–85.

———. "Prevalence of Psychiatric Disorders in Metropolitan Old Age and Nursing Homes." *Journal of American Geriatrics Society* 10 (1962):181–85.

———. *Aging and Organic Brain Syndrome*. New York: Health Learning Systems, 1974.

Goldsmith, J. "Community Crime Prevention and the Elderly: A Segmental Approach." *Crime Prevention Review*, California State Attorney General's Office, July 1975, p. 19.

Goldsmith, J. and Tomas, N. "Crime Against the Elderly: A Continuing National Problem." *Aging* 236–237 (July-August 1974).

Goldsmith, S. and Goldsmith, J. "Crime, the Aging, and Public Policy." *Perspective on Aging* (May-June 1975):16–19.

Goldstein, G. and Shelley, C. "Similarities and Differences Between Psychological Deficit in Aging and Brain Damage." *Journal of Gerontology* 30 (1975):448–55.

Gordon, G. *Role Theory and Illness: A Social Perspective*. New Haven: College & University Press, 1966.

Gregory, R. "A Survey of Residents in Five Nursing and Rest Homes in Cumberland County, North Carolina." *Journal of American Geriatrics Society* 18 (1970):501–6.

Gubrium, J. and Ksander, M. "On Multiple Realities and Reality Orientation." *Gerontologist* 15 (1975):142–45.

Gunter, L. "Students' Attitudes toward Geriatric Nursing." *Nursing Outlook* 19 (1971):466–69.

Gurian, B. and Scherl, D. "A Community Focused Model of Mental Health Services for the Elderly." *Journal of Geriatric Psychiatry* 5 (1972):77–78.

Hackett, T.; Cassem, N.; and Wishnie, H. "The Coronary-Care Unit: An Appraisal of Its Psychologic Hazards." *New England Journal of Medicine* 279 (1968):1365–70.

Harmon, D. "Geriatric Nutrition." In *Quick Reference to Clinical Nutrition*, edited by S. Halpern. Philadelphia: Lippincott, 1979.

Harris, C. and Ivory, P. "An Outcome Evaluation of Reality Orientation Therapy with Geriatric Patients in a State Mental Hospital." *Gerontologist* 16 (1976):496–503.

Harris, L. and Associates. *The Myth and Reality of Aging in America*. Washington: National Council on the Aging, 1975.

Hausknecht, M. *The Joiners*. New York: Bedminster Press, 1962.

Havice, D. "Old Age: The Possibility of Enlightenment." *Soundings* (Spring 1974):70–79.

Havighurst, R. and Sacher, G. "Prospects of Lengthening Life and Vigor." In *Extending the Human Life Span: Social Policy and Social Ethics*, edited by B. Neugarten and R. Havighurst. Washington, D.C.: National Science Foundation, 1977.

Hayflick, L. "Perspectives on Human Longevity." In *Extending the Human Life Span: Social Policy and Social Ethics*, edited by B. Neugarten and R. Havighurst. Washington, D.C.: National Science Foundation, 1977.

Hearn, L. *Japan: An Interpretation*. Rutland, Vt.: Charles E. Tuttle, 1955.

Hellebrandt, F. "Comment: The Senile Dement in Our Midst: A Look at the Other Side of the Coin." *Gerontologist* 18 (1978):67–70.

Hendricks, J. and Hendricks, C. *Aging in Mass Society: Myths and Realities*. Cambridge, Mass.: Winthrop, 1977.

Henry, W. "The Theory of Intrinsic Disengagement." In *Age with a Future*, edited by P. Hanson. Philadelphia: Davis, 1964.

Herbert, V. "Facts and Fictions about Megavitamin Therapy." *Resident and Staff Physician*, 1978, pp. 43–50.

Heyman, D. "Does a Wife Retire?" *Gerontologist* 10 (1970):54–56.

Hindelang, M. *Criminal Victimization in Eight American Cities*. Law Enforcement Assistance Administration, Washington, D.C.: U.S. Government Printing Office, 1975.

Hochschild, A. *The Unexpected Community*. Englewood Cliffs, N.J.: Prentice-Hall, 1973.

———. "Disengagement Theory: A Critique and Proposal." *American Sociological Review* 40 (1975):553–69.

Holland, J. "The Krebiozen Story: Is Cancer Quackery Dead?" *Proceedings*, Third National Congress on Medical Quackery, Chicago, 1966.

Holmes, D. and Jorgenson, B. "Do Personality and Social Psychologists Study Men More Than Women?" *Government Reports Announcement*, 25 December 1971.

Holmes, T. and Rahe, R. "The Social Readjustment Rating Scale." *Journal of Psychosomatic Research* 11 (1967):213–18.

Holzman, J. and Beck, J. "Palmore's Facts on Aging Quiz: A Reappraisal." *Gerontologist* 19 (1979):116–20.

Horn, J. and Cattell, R. "Refinement and Test of the Theory of Fluid and Crystallized Intelligence." *Journal of Educational Psychology* 57 (1966):253–70.

———. "Age Differences in Fluid and Crystallized Intelligence." *Acta Psychologica* 26 (1967):107–29.

Horn, J. and Donaldson, G. "On the Myth of Intellectual Decline in Adulthood." *American Psychologist* 31 (1976):701–9.

———. "Faith Is Not Enough: Response to the Baltes-Schaie Claim that Intelligence Does Not Wane." *American Psychologist* 32 (1977):369–73.

Hoyer, W.; Labouvie, G.; and Baltes, P. "Modification of Response Speed and Intellectual Performance in the Elderly." *Human Development* 16 (1973): 233–42.

Hudson, R. "Death, Dying and the Zealous Phase." *Annals of Internal Medicine* 88 (1978):696–702.

Hughes, E. *Men and Their Work*. Glencoe, Ill.: Free Press, 1958.

Isaacs, B.; Livingston, L.; and Neville, Y. *Survival of the Unfittest: A Study of Geriatric Patients in Glasgow*. London and Boston: Routledge & Kegan Paul, 1972.

Jackson, J. "Negro Aged: Toward Needed Research in Social Gerontology." *Gerontologist* 11 (1971):52–57.

Japan Census Bureau. *1965 Population Census*. Tokyo: Census Bureau, 1965.

Jarvick, L. and Russell, D. "Anxiety, Aging and the Third Emergency Reaction." *Journal of Gerontology* 34 (1979):197–200.

Kahn, R.; Goldfarb, A.; Pollack, M.; and Peck, A. "Brief Objective Measure for the Determination of Mental Status in the Aged." *American Journal of Psychiatry* 117 (1960):326.

Kalish, R. "Of Social Values and the Dying: A Defense of Disengagement." *Family Coordinator* 21 (1972):81–94.

———. Review of *The Myth and Reality of Aging in America*, by L. Harris. Washington, D.C., National Council on Aging, 1975, in *The Gerontologist*, 15 (1975):564–65.

———. "The New Ageism and the Failure Models: A Polemic." *Gerontologist* 19 (1979):398–407.

————. *Death, the Process of Dying and Grief.* Monterey, Calif.: Brooks/Cole, forthcoming.

Kammerman, S. and Kahn, A. *Not for the Poor Alone: European Social Services.* Philadelphia: Temple University Press, 1975.

Kastenbaum, R. and Aisenberg, R. *The Psychology of Death.* New York: Springer, 1972.

Kastenbaum, R. and Candy, S. "The Four Percent Fallacy: A Methodological and Empirical Critique of Extended Care Facility Program Statistics. *Aging and Human Development* 4 (1973):15–21.

Kimmel, D. *Adulthood and Aging.* New York: Wiley, 1974.

Kleban, M.; Lawton, M.; Brody, E.; and Moss, M. "Characteristics of Mentally Impaired Profiting from Individualized Treatment." *Journal of Gerontology* 30 (1975):90–96.

————. "Behavior Observation of Mentally Impaired: Those Who Decline and Those Who Do Not." *Journal of Gerontology* 31 (1976):333–39.

Klemmack, D. "Comment: An Examination of Palmore's Facts on Aging Quiz." *Gerontologist* 18 (1978):403–6.

Kline, C. "The Socialization Process of Women: Implications for a Successful Theory of Aging." *Gerontologist* 15 (1975):486–92.

Knowles, J. *Doing Better and Feeling Worse: Health in the United States.* New York: Norton, 1977.

Kossoris, M. "Absenteeism and Injury Experience of Older Workers." *Monthly Labor Review* 67 (1948):16–19.

Kramer, C. and Kramer, J. "Establishing a Therapeutic Community in the Nursing Home." *Professional Nursing Home* (September, October, November 1966; January, February, April 1967).

Kreps, J. "Career Options After Fifty: Suggested Research." *Gerontologist* 11 (1971):4–8.

Kübler-Ross, E. *On Death and Dying.* New York: Macmillan, 1969.

————. *Death: The Final Stage of Growth.* Englewood Cliffs, N.J.: Prentice-Hall, 1975.

Lapham, L. "The Easy Chair: Perspective on Flight." *Harpers Magazine* 257 (August 1978):12–14.

Leaf, A. "Everyday is a Gift When You Are Over 100." *National Geographic* 148 (January 1973a):93–117.

————. "Getting Old." *Scientific American* 229 (1973b):45–52.

————. "Statement Regarding the Purportedly Longevous Peoples of Vilcabamba. Mimeographed, n.d.

Lerner, M. *America as a Civilization: Life and Thought in the United States Today.* New York: Simon & Schuster, 1957.

Lieberman, M. "Relocation Research and Social Policy." *Gerontologist* 14 (1974):494–501. Also in *Communities and Environmental Policy,* edited by J. Gubrium. New York: Charles C Thomas, 1974.

Lieberman, M. and Coplan, A. "Distance from Death as a Variable in the Study of Aging." *Developmental Psychology* 2 (1970):71–84.

Lieberman, M. and Mullan, J. "Does Help Help? The Adaptive Consequences of Obtaining Help from Professionals and Social Networks." *American Journal of Community Psychology* 6 (1978):499–517.

Lin, N.; Simeone, R.; Enesel, W.; and Kaw, W. "Social Support, Stressful Life Events, and Illness: A Model and Empirical Test. *Journal of Health and Social Behavior* 20 (1979):108–19.

Lopata, H. "The Life Cycle of the Social Role of the Housewife." *Sociology and Social Research* 51 (1966):5–22.

———. *Occupation: Housewife*. New York and London: Oxford University Press, 1971a.

———. "Widows as a minority group." *Gerontologist* 11 (1971b):22–27.

———. *Widowhood in an American City*. Boston: Schenkman, 1972.

Lopata, H. and Steinhart, F. "Work Histories of American Urban Women." *Gerontologist* 11 (1971):27–36.

Lowenthal, M. and Berkman, P. *Aging and Mental Disorder in San Francisco*. San Francisco: Jossey-Bass, 1967.

Lozier, J. and Althouse, R. "Retirement to the Porch in Rural Appalachia." *Aging and Human Development* 6 (1975):7–16.

McCord, A. Review of E. Palmore, *The Honorable Elders*. *Sociology* 3 (February 1976):68–69.

McKinney, F.; Lorian, R.; and Zax, M. *Effective Behavior and Human Development*. New York: Macmillan, 1976.

McPherson, F. and Fox, M. "Treatment of Breast Cancer." In *Costs, Risks, and Benefits of Surgery*, edited by J. Bunker, B. Barnes, and F. Moestellar. Oxford: Oxford University Press, 1977.

Maddox, G. "Disengagement Theory: A Critical Evaluation." *Gerontologist* 9 (1969):80–83.

Maddox, G. and Douglas, E. "Aging and Individual Differences." *Journal of Gerontology* 29 (1974):555–63.

Malinchak, A. and Wright, D. "The Scope of Victimization of the Elderly." *Aging* 281–282 (March-April 1978):12–16.

Marmor, T. and Kudrle, R. "The Health Care Crisis." Paper presented at a symposium on political and community problems in mental health care, Northern Illinois University, 23 April 1975.

Marnell, G. "Comparative Correctional Systems: United States and Sweden." *Criminal Law Bulletin* 8 (1972):748–60.

Martin, C. "Lavender Rose or Gray Panther?" *Aging* 285–286 (1978):28–30.

Masters, W. and Johnson, V. *Human Sexual Response*. Boston: Little, Brown, 1966.

Mazess, R. and Forman, S. "Longevity and Age Exaggeration in Vilcabamba." *Journal of Gerontology* 34 (1979):94–98.

Meacher, M. *Taken for a Ride*. London: Longman, 1972.

Mead, M. *Sex and Temperament in Three Primitive Societies*. New York: William Morrow & Co., 1935.

———. *Male and Female: A Study of the Sexes in a Changing World*. New York: William Morrow & Co., 1949.

Medvedev, Z. "Caucasus and Altay Longevity: A Biological or Social Problem?" *Gerontologist* 14 (1974):381–86.

Metropolitan Life Insurance Company. *Statistical Bulletin* 60 (1979).

Miller, D.; Lowenstein, R.; and Winston, R. "Physicians' Attitudes Toward the Ill Aged and Nursing Homes." *Journal of American Geriatrics Society* 24 (1976):498–505.

Miller, S. "The Social Dilemma of the Aging Leisure Participant." In *Older People and Their Social World*, edited by A. Rose and W. Peterson. Philadelphia: Davis, 1965.

Mills, J. "Attitudes of Undergraduate Students Concerning Geriatric Patients." *American Journal of Occupational Therapy* 26 (1972):200–3.

Ministry of Health and Welfare. *Tokyo Steps Up Social Welfare*, 1974.

Morris, N. "Lessons from the Adult Educational Correctional System of Sweden." *Federal Probation* 30 (December 1966).

Morris, R. "Aging and the Field of Social Work." In *Aging and Society: Vol. 2 Aging and the Professions*, edited by M. Riley, J. Riley, and M. Johnson. New York: Russell Sage, 1969, pp. 3–13.

Mueller, C. "Notes on the Repression of Communicative Behavior." In *Recent Sociology, No. 2: Patterns of Communicative Behavior*, edited by H. Dreitzel. London: Macmillan, 1970.

Mulvey, M. "Psychological and Sociological Factors in Prediction of Career Patterns of Women." *Genetic Psychological Monographs*, No. 68, 1963.

Myers, R. "An Investigation of the Age of an Alleged Centenarian." *Demography* 15 (1978):235–36.

Nagorny, A.; Nikitin, V.; and Bulankin, J. *Problems of Aging and Longevity*. Moscow: Publishing House Medicina, 1963.

Nakane, C. *Japanese Society*. Berkeley: University of California Press, 1972.

National Center for Health Statistics. *Health Characteristics of Persons with Chronic Activity Limitation*, series 10, no. 112. Washington, D.C.: U.S. Government Printing Office, 1974.

National Safety Council. *Accident Facts*. Chicago: National Safety Council, 1976.

Neugarten, B., ed. "Aging in the Year 2000." *Gerontologist* 15, 1975.

Neugarten, B.; Crotty, W.; and Tobin, S. "Personality Types in an Aged Population." In *Personality in Middle and Later Life*, edited by B. Neugarten. New York: Atherton, 1964.

Neugarten, B. and Havighurst, R., eds. *Social Policy, Social Ethics and the Aging Society*. Washington, D.C.: National Science Foundation, 1976.

———. *Extending the Human Life Span: Social Policy and Social Ethics*. Washington, D.C.: National Science Foundation, 1977.

Neugarten, B.; Wood, V.; Krains, R.; and Loomis, B. "Womens' Attitudes toward the Menopause." *Vita Humana* 6 (1963):140-51.

Noyes, R. and Kletti, R. "Depersonalization in the Face of Life-Threatening Danger: A Description." *Psychiatry* 39 (1976):19–27.

Office of the Prime Minister. *Public Opinion Survey About Problems of Old Age*. Tokyo: Office of the Prime Minister, 1973.

Osmond, H. and Siegler, M. "The Dying Role: Its Clinical Importance." *Alabama Journal of Medical Sciences* 13 (1976):313–17.

Ostfeld, A.; Smith, C.; and Stotsky, B. "The Systematic Use of Procaine in the Treatment of the Elderly: A Review." *Journal of American Geriatrics Society* 25 (1977):11–20.

Palmore, E. "Work Experiences and Earnings of the Aged." *Social Security Bulletin* 27 (1964):3–15.

——. "Differences in the Retirement Patterns of Men and Women." *Gerontologist* 5 (1965):4–8.

——. "Sociological Aspects of Aging." In *Behavior and Adaptation in Later Life*, edited by E. Busse and E. Pfeiffer. Boston: Little, Brown, 1969.

——. "Health Practices and Illness among the Aged." *Gerontologist* 10 (1970):313–16.

——. "Compulsory vs. Flexible Retirement: Issues and Facts." *Gerontologist* 12 (1972):343–48.

——. "Ageism Compared to Racism and Sexism." *Journal of Gerontology* 28 (1973):363–69.

——. *Normal Aging, Vol. 2*. Durham, N.C.: Duke University Press, 1974a.

——. "The Brighter Side of Four Score and Ten." *Gerontologist* 14 (1974b):136–37.

——. "What Can the U.S. Learn from Japan about Aging?" *Gerontologist* 15 (1975a):64–67.

——. *The Honorable Elders*. Durham, N.C.: Duke University Press, 1975b.

——. "The Future Status of the Aged." *Gerontologist* 16 (1976a):297–302.

——. "Total Chance of Institutionalization in the Aged." *Gerontologist* 16 (1976b):504–7.

——. "Facts on Aging: A Short Quiz." *Gerontologist* 17 (1978):315–20.

Palmore, E. and Luickart, F. "Health and Social Factors Related to Life Satisfaction." *Journal of Health and Social Behavior* 13 (1977):68–80.

Parsons, T. *The Social System*. Glencoe, Ill.: Free Press, 1951.

Penzias, A. "The Cosmic Background: Interview with Arnold Penzias," by E. Oxford. *Bell Telephone Magazine* 58 (February 1979):25–27.

Peterson, O. "Myocardial Infarction: Unit Care or Home Care?" *New England Journal of Medicine* 28 (1978):259–61.

Pfeiffer, E. "A Short Portable Mental Status Questionnaire for the Assessment of Organic Brain Deficit in Elderly Patients. *Journal of the American Geriatrics Society* 23 (1975):433–41.

Pitot, H. "Carcinogenesis and Aging: Two Related Phenomena?" *American Journal of Pathology* 87 (1977).

Pizhelauri, G. and Lugovoi, V. "Zones of Longevity in Georgia." In *Questions of Gerontology and Geriatrics*, edited by N. Gorev. Leningrad: Medical Publishing House, 1962.

Plath, D. "Japan: The After Years." In *Aging and Modernization*, edited by D. Cowgill and L. Holmes. New York: Appleton-Century-Crofts, 1972.

Pope, C. and Feyerherm, W. "A Review of Recent Trends: The Effects of Crime on the Elderly." *The Police Chief*, February 1976, p. 29.

Rabkin, J. and Struening, E. "Life Events, Stress, and Illness. *Science*, 3 December 1976, pp. 1013–20.

Rahe, R.; Bennett, L.; Romo, M.; Silatenen, P.; and Arthur, R. "Subjects' Recent Life Changes and Coronary Heart Disease in Finland." *American Journal of Psychiatry* 130 (1973):1222–26.

Rather, D. "CBS Evening News with Dan Rather," 28 February 1976.

Rawlings, M. *Beyond Death's Door*. Nashville: Nelson, 1978.

Reichard, S.; Livson, F.; and Peterson, P. *Aging and Personality*. New York: Wiley, 1962.

Riegel, K. and Riegel, R. "A Study of the Drop-Out Rates in Longitudinal Research on Aging and the Prediction of Death." *Journal of Personality and Social Psychology* 5 (1967):342, 348.

———. "Development, Drop and Death." *Developmental Psychology* 6 (1972): 306–19.

Reinhart, G. Personal communication.

Reisman, D. *The Lonely Crowd: A Study of the Changing American Character*. New Haven: Yale University Press, 1950.

Riley, M. Review of E. Palmore, *The Honorable Elders*. *Social Forces* 55 (1976):564–65.

Riley, M. and Foner, A. *Aging and Society, Vol 1*. New York: Russell Sage Foundation, 1968.

Roazen, P. *Freud and His Followers*. New York: Knopf, 1975.

Robbins, W. *The American Food Scandal*. New York: William Morrow, 1974.

Rosow, I. "Retirement Leisure and Social Status." In *Proceedings of Seminars, 1965–1969*, edited by F. Jeffers. Duke University Council on Human Development, 1969, pp. 149–57.

———. "The Aged in Post-Affluent Society." *Gerontology* (Israel) 1 (1975): 9–22.

Rubin, R.; Gunderson, E.; and Dall, R. "Life Stress and Illness Patterns in the U.S. Navy—I. Environmental Variables and Illness Onset in an Attack Carrier's Crew." *Archives of Environmental Health* 19 (1969):740.

Russell, B. *Philosophy*. New York: Norton, 1927.

———. *A History of Western Philosophy*. New York: Clarion Books, Simon & Schuster, 1945.

Sacher, G. "Life-Table Modification and Life Prolongation." In *Handbook of the Biology of Aging*, edited by J. Birren, L. Hayflick, and C. Finch. New York: Van Nostrand, 1977.

Sandok, B. "Organic Brain Syndrome." In *Comprehensive Textbook of Psychiatry, Vol. 1*, edited by A. Freedman, H. Kaplan, and B. Sandock. Baltimore: Williams and Wilkins, 1975.

Saunders, C. "The Last Stage of Life." *American Journal of Nursing* 65 (1965):70–75.

———. "The Moment of Truth." In *Death and Dying*, edited by L. Pearson. Cleveland: Case-Western Reserve University Press, 1969.

———. "Words vs. Deeds." In *The Sociologist as Detective: An Introduction to Research Methods*, edited by W. Saunders. New York: Praeger, 1976.

Schaie, K. "Translations in Gerontology: From Lab to Life: Intellectual Functioning." *American Psychologist* 29 (1974):802–7.

————. "A General Model for the Study of Developmental Problems." *Psychological Bulletin* 64 (1965):92–107.

Schaie, K. and Baltes, P. "Some Faith Helps to see the Trees: A Final Comment on the Horn and Donaldson Myth of the Baltes-Schaie Position on Adult Intelligence." *American Psychologist* 32 (1977):1118–20.

Schooler, K. "The Relationship Between Social Interaction and Morale of the Elderly as a Function of Environmental Characteristics." *Gerontologist* 9 (1969):25–29.

Selye, H. *The Stress of Life*. New York: McGraw-Hill, 1956.

Serrill, M. "Profile/Sweden." *Corrections Magazine* 3 (June 1977):11–34.

Settin, J. "Comment: Some Thoughts about Diseases Presenting as Senility." *Gerontologist* 18 (1978):71–72.

Sheldon, J. *Social Medicine of Old Age*. London: Oxford University Press, 1947.

Shock, N. "The Physiology of Aging." *Scientific American* 206 (1962):100–10.

Siegel, S. "Some Demographic Aspects of Aging in the U.S." In *Epidemiology of Aging*, edited by M. Ostfeld and D. Gibson. DHEW Publication (NIH), Washington, D.C.: U.S. Government Printing Office, 1974, pp. 75–111.

Simmons, L. *The Role of the Aged in Primitive Society*. New Haven: Yale University Press, 1945.

Sleisenger, M. and Fordtran, J. *Gastrointestinal Disease: Pathology, Diagnosis, Management*. Philadelphia: W. B. Saunders, 1978.

Sommers, T. "The Compounding Impact of Age on Sex." *Civil Rights Digest* 7 (1974):3–9.

Sontag, S. "The Double Standard of Aging." *Saturday Review of the Society*, 23 September 1972, pp. 29–38.

Spaskukozki, Y.; Barchenki, L.; and Genis, E. *Longevity and Physiological Aging*. Kiev: State Medical Publishing House, 1963.

Spence, D. and Feigenbaum, E. "Medical Students' Attitudes toward the Geriatric Patient." *Journal of Gerontology* 16 (1968):976–83.

Steinman, A. "A Study of the Concept of the Feminine Role of 51 Middle-Class American Families." *Genetic Psychological Monographs*, no. 67, 1963.

Stotsky, B. "Nursing Homes: A Review." *American Journal of Psychiatry* 3 (1966):249–58.

Strehler, B. "A New Age for Aging." *Natural History* 82 (February 1973):9–18, 82–85.

Streib, G. "Disengagement Theory in Sociocultural Perspective." In *New Thoughts on Old Age*, edited by R. Kastenbaum. New York: Springer, 1964, pp. 69–76.

Streib, G. and Schneider, C. *Retirement in American Society: Impact and Process*. Ithaca: Cornell University Press, 1971.

Taylor, P. and Ingrasci, R. "Out of the Body: An Interview with Elizabeth Kübler-Ross." *New Age*, November 1977.

Thurnwald, R. Review of M. Mead, "Sex and Temperament in Three Primitive Societies." *American Anthropologist* 38 (1936):663–67.

Tighe, J. H. "A Survey of Crime against the Elderly." *Police Chief*, February 1977, p. 19.

Time Magazine. "High Hoax: Those Not So Old Ecuadorians," 27 March 1978, pp. 87–88.

Tobin, S. and Thompson, D. "The 'countability' paradox of social programs." Paper presented at International Congress of Gerontology, Jerusalem, Israel, June 1975.

U.S., Commerce Department, Bureau of the Census, Special Subject Report. *Persons in Institutions and Other Group Quarters*. Washington, D.C.: U.S. Government Printing Office, 1970.

U.S., Commerce Department, Bureau of the Census, Current Population Survey. *Projections of the Population of the U.S. by Age and Sex: 1975–2000*, series P-25, #541. Washington, D.C.: U.S. Government Printing Office, 1975.

U.S., Congress, *Congressional Record*, 94th Cong., 1st sess., 1975, 121, 516613, 516738.

U.S., Congress, House, Subcommittee on Federal, State and Community Services of the House Select Committee on Aging, *Crime against the Elderly*, 94th Cong., 2d sess., 13 December 1976.

U.S., Congress, House, Subcommittee on Housing and Consumer Interests of the House Select Committee on Aging, *Elderly Crime Victimization* (Federal Law Enforcement Agencies—L.E.A.A. and F.B.I.), 94th Cong., 2d sess., 12–13 April 1976, p. 24.

U.S., Congress, House, Subcommittee on Housing and Consumer Interests of the House Select Committee on Aging, *In Search of Security: A National Perspective on Elderly Crime Victimization*, 95th Cong., 1st sess., April 1977.

U.S., Congress, Senate, Committee on the Judiciary. *Our Nation's Schools' Report Card: "A" in School Violence and Vandalism*. Washington, D.C.: U.S. Government Printing Office, 1975.

U.S., Congress, Senate, Special Committee on Aging, *Hearings before the Subcommittee on Housing for the Elderly*, 92d Cong., 1st sess., October 1971.

U.S., Congress, Senate, Special Committee on Aging, *Hearings before the Subcommittee on Housing for the Elderly*, 92d Cong., 2d sess., 11 August 1972, p. 481; October 1972, p. 542.

U.S., Congress, Senate, Subcommittee on Retirement and the Individual of the Special Committee on Aging, *The Federal Role in Encouraging Preretirement Counselling and New Work: Lifetime Patterns*, 91st Cong., 1st sess., 25 July 1969.

U.S., Congress, Senate, Subcommittee of the Senate Special Committee on Aging. *Hearings before the Subcommittee on Housing for the Elderly*, 92d Cong., 1st sess., October 1971. Washington, D.C.: U.S. Government Printing Office, 1971.

U.S. Congress, Senate, Special Committee on Aging. *Report on Nursing Home Care in the United States*, December 1974, Supporting Paper #1. Washington, D.C.: U.S. Government Printing Office, 1974.

U.S., Department of Health, Education and Welfare, Health Care Financing Administration, Office of Policy, Planning and Research, *Research and Statistics Note,* June 1978.

U.S., Department of Health, Education and Welfare, Social Security Administration, Office of Research and Statistics. *The 1967 National Survey of Institutionalized Adults: Residents of Long-Term Care Institutions.* DHEW Publication (SSA) 75-11803, 1974.

U.S., Department of Justice, Law Enforcement Assistance Administration. *Criminal Victimization in the United States: A National Crime Panel Survey Report.* Washington, D.C.: U.S. Government Printing Office, May 1975.

Van Gennep, A. *The Rite of Passage.* London: Routledge & Kegan Paul, 1960.

Vital Health Statistics. *Chronic Conditions and Impairments of Nursing Home Residents.* DHEW Publication (HSM), Washington, D.C.: U.S. Government Printing Office, 73–1704, 1973.

Vital Health Statistics. *Life Tables, Vol. 2, Section 5, 1975.* Washington, D.C.: National Center for Health Statistics, 1977.

Wain, J. *Samuel Johnson—A Biography.* New York: Viking, 1975.

Wasserman, J. *The World's Illusion.* New York: Popular Library, 1976.

Wells, C. "Dementia Reconsidered." *Archives of General Psychiatry* 26 (1972):385–88.

Wershow, H. "The Balance of Mental Health and Regression, as Expressed in the Literature on Chronic Illness and Disability." *Social Service Review* 37 (1963):193–200.

———. "The Older Jews of Albany Park: Some Aspects of a Subculture of the Aged and its Interaction with a Gerontological Research Project." *Gerontologist* 4 (1964):198–202.

———. "Aging in the Israeli Kibbutz." *Gerontologist* 9 (1969):300–4.

———. "Aging in the Israeli Kibbutz: Some Further Investigation." *Aging and Human Development* 4 (1973a):211–27.

———. "Mankind: A Maladjusted Species?" *Ecology of Foods and Nutrition* 2 (1973b):69–72.

———. "The Four Percent Fallacy: Some Further Evidence and Policy Implications." *Gerontologist* 16 (1976):52–55.

———. "Setting Priorities in Health and Welfare Services." *Health and Social Work* 1 (1977a):6–24.

———. "A Pilot Study of Black and White Nursing Home Patients in Birmingham and Rural Alabama." Unpublished, 1977b.

———. "Comment: Reality Orientation for the Gerontologist: Some Thoughts about Senility." *Gerontologist* 17 (1977c):297–302.

———. "The Outer Limits of the Welfare State: Discrimination, Racism, and Their Effect on Human Services." *Aging and Human Development* 10 (1979–1980):63–75.

Wershow, H. and Reinhart, G. "Life Change and Hospitalization—A Heretical View." *Journal of Psychomatic Research* 18 (1974):393–401.

White House Conference on Aging. *Toward a National Policy on Aging, Vol. 2.* Washington, D.C.: U.S. Government Printing Office, 1973.

Wilder, T. *Our Town.* New York: Coward, McCann & Geoghegan, 1938.

Wilensky, H. "The Politics of Taxation: America in World Perspective." In *Taxation: Myth and Realities,* edited by G. Break and B. Wallin. Menlo Park, Calif. and Reading, Mass.: Addison-Wesley, 1978.

Winston, E. "The Alleged Lack of Mental Disease among Primitive Groups." *American Anthropologist* 36 (1934):236–37.

Women's Bureau. *1969 Handbook on Women Workers.* Bulletin no. 294, Washington, D.C.: U.S. Department of Labor, 1969.

Woodruff, D. and Birren, J., eds. *Aging: Scientific Perspective and Social Issues.* New York: Van Nostrand, 1975.

Index

Index